PRAISE FOR BRENDAN BRAZIER

"Brendan's plant-based nutrition concepts, combined with his innovative holistic approach to training, will get you in the best mental and physical shape of your life. *Thrive Fitness* is truly the way to unleash your full potential!"

    —Venus Williams

"I am forever grateful to Brendan . . . I have noticed increased energy and more-restful sleep. My desire for sugar and salt is waning."

    —Hugh Jackman

"When I train and need to be at my very best physically and mentally, I turn to Brendan. I highly recommend his book *The Thrive Diet*."

    —Brian Roberts, second baseman, Baltimore Orioles,
      two-time MLB All-Star

"*Thrive Fitness* is the blueprint for achieving optimum performance and living a clean and healthy existence. I've incorporated all of Brendan's principles into my training, and I've never felt healthier and stronger."

    —Mike Bryan, World No. 1–ranked doubles tennis player
      (with his brother Bob); winner of Wimbledon, US Open,
      French Open, Australian Open; Olympic gold medalist

"*The Thrive Diet* was an absolute game changer for me in regards to knowledge about eating for performance and overall healthy living. Brazier's vision of plant-based nutrition not only helped me become a better and healthier athlete but has inspired me to help others make better choices when it comes to fueling the body."

    —Kenny Florian, former elite UFC fighter, color commentator for
      UFC Fight Night on Fox

"*The Thrive Diet* has been one of my fundamental and most valuable tools in helping me dive into the world of proper nutrition, fitness and all around wellness. I'm so thankful for Brendan sharing his sea of knowledge through this book . . . a must read for anyone ready to take back their life!"
—Rebecca Soni, six-time Olympic medalist, swimming

"Brendan gets it! His nutritional approach is what supercharges results."
—Tony Horton, creator of P90X, the world's bestselling workout program

"When world-class athletes want to get even better, Brendan is the man who gets the call."
—Brendon Burchard, *New York Times* bestselling author of *The Charge*

"As our head of nutrition, Brendan's implementation of purpose-driven nutrition has allowed our pro cycling team to meet the demands of grueling training better than ever before."
—Matt Johnson, President of Cannondale-Garmin Pro Cycling Team and founder of The Feed

"Brendan's systematic approach to performance plant-based nutrition has helped me to reduce inflammation, speed my recovery, and has boosted my overall performance. The recipes are delicious!"
—Mike Zigomanis, NHL player and member of the 2009 Stanley Cup champion Pittsburgh Penguins

"This guide is what your plant-based kitchen is missing. You're going to feel better, and you're going to enjoy every bite. Oh, and in case you were wondering: You're not going to miss the meat."
—Angela Haupt, senior editor of *U.S. News & World Report*

"Brendan's commitment to the study of plant-based nutrition and research makes for a wonderful cookbook."
—Joe Hogarty, Baltimore Orioles strength and conditioning coach

"*Thrive Energy Cookbook* is a must-have for gourmets and athletes alike."
—Sean Hyson, C.S.C.S., Group Training Director for *Men's Fitness* and
Muscle & Fitness magazines

"Brendan makes learning to eat healthier enjoyable, and his approach to better health simply makes sense. Take the leap and eat the 'Thrive' way."
—Terri MacLeod, *Access Hollywood*

"*Whole Foods To Thrive* offers a diet that's good for you and the planet."
—*The Washington Post*

"*The Thrive Diet* focuses on vegan foods that help fuel your way to uber athleticism."
—*CNN*

"The *Thrive* diet feeds your body all the nutrients it needs without empty calories and with minimal stress."
—*Chicago Tribune*

"Brendan's knowledge is second to none. I read *The Thrive Diet* and was enthralled that after reading so many books and meeting with so many experts, Brendan was able to explain his thoughts on nutrition in such a clear and insightful way . . . I only hope my competition doesn't read this book until after I'm done competing."
—Simon Whitfield, Olympic silver (triathlon, Beijing 2008) and gold
(triathlon, Sydney 2000) medalist

"*The Thrive Diet* is packed with invaluable information that can assist anyone at any level. I wish Brendan all the best."
—Bruny Surin, Olympic gold medalist (4x100 meter relay, Atlanta 1996)

"The guidelines in *The Thrive Diet* work to help maintain your body's optimal health level whether you're a world-class athlete, a 9 to 5'er, or a stay-at-home mom . . . There's no other resource like it out there."
—Mac Danzig, Ultimate Fighter 6 Champion

"*The Thrive Diet* is ideal for dieters who want to reduce their carbon foot-print and get healthy at the same time."
　　—*The Library Journal*

"I can't say enough good things about *The Thrive Diet* and honestly be-lieve that every athlete, trainer, or coach owes it to themselves to read it."
　　—Jason Ferruggia, Chief Training Advisor to *Men's Fitness* magazine

"*The Thrive Diet* is an authoritative guide to outstanding performance, not just in top-level athletics, but in day-to-day life . . . This book sets aside the myths that have held many people back, and provides a state-of-the-art program for top health."
　　—Neal D. Barnard, M.D., President, Physicians Committee for
　　Responsible Medicine

"*The Thrive Diet* is a life-changing book! The nutritional approach that Brendan has created is amazing, and all backed with powerful facts. If you want to reduce stress, feel great, and attain peak performance, get *The Thrive Diet*!"
　　—Jon Hinds, former strength coach of the LA Clippers, advisor to MLB
　　and NFL teams

"*The Thrive Diet* is an excellent source of information for anyone wanting to improve their own health by eating a whole-food, plant-based diet."
　　—Mitzi Dulan, R.D., CSSD, Team Sports Nutritionist: Kansas City Chiefs
　　and Kansas City Royals

"Brendan Brazier's *The Thrive Diet* will increase the micronutrient density of your eating style and enable you to live longer, live healthier and thrive."
　　—Joel Fuhrman, M.D., bestselling author of *Eat to Live* and *Eat for Health*

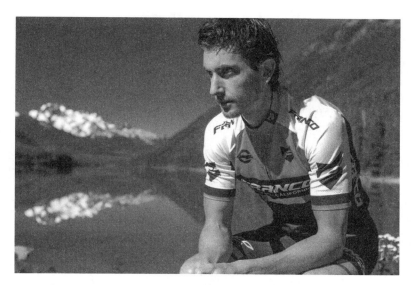

Brendan Brazier is the international bestselling author of the *Thrive* book series, and co-founder and formulator of Vega. He is recognized as one of the world's foremost authorities on plant-based, performance nutrition, and is head of Nutrition for the Cannondale-Garmin Pro Cycling Team and nutrition consultant to a number of NHL, MLB, NFL, MLS, UFC, and Olympic athletes. He is a former professional Ironman triathlete and two-time Canadian 50km ultra-marathon champion.

www.brendanbrazier.com
T: @brendan_brazier
I: @brendanbrazier
F: www.facebook.com/brendanbrazier

ALSO BY BRENDAN BRAZIER

The Thrive Diet: The Whole Foods Way to Losing
Weight, Reducing Stress, and Staying Healthy for Life

Whole Foods to Thrive:
Nutrient-Dense Plant-Based Recipes for Peak Health

Thrive Energy Cookbook:
150 Functional, Plant-Based Whole Food Recipes

SECOND EDITION

THRIVE FITNESS

THE PROGRAM FOR PEAK MENTAL & PHYSICAL STRENGTH
FUELED BY CLEAN, PLANT-BASED, WHOLE FOOD RECIPES

BRENDAN BRAZIER

PENGUIN

an imprint of Penguin Canada, a division of
Penguin Random House Canada Limited

Published in Penguin paperback by Penguin Canada, 2015
Simultaneously published in the United States by Da Capo Press,
44 Farnsworth Street, 3rd Floor, Boston, MA 02210

1 2 3 4 5 6 7 8 9 10 (RRD)

Exercise photos: Donovan Jenkins and Alex Richardson
Diagrams and nutrition icons: Tommy Heiden

Dan Piraro's *Bizarro* cartoon used with permission

The information in this book is true and complete to the best of our knowledge.
This book is intended only as an informative guide for those wishing to know more about
health issues. In no way is this book intended to replace, countermand, or conflict with the advice
given to you by your own physician. The ultimate decision concerning care should be made between you
and your doctor. We strongly recommend you follow his or her advice. Information in this book
is general and is offered with no guarantees on the part of the author or Penguin Canada.
The author and publisher disclaim all liability in connection with the use of this book.

Text design: Trish Wilkinson
Cover design: Alex Camlin
Cover photograph: Rob Campbell

Manufactured in the U.S.A.

Library and Archives Canada Cataloguing in Publication

Brazier, Brendan, author
Thrive fitness : the program for peak mental & physical strength fueled
by clean, plant-based, whole food recipes / Brendan Brazier.—Second edition.

Includes bibliographical references and index.
ISBN 978-0-14-319809-3 (paperback)
1. Physical fitness. 2. Health. 3. Nutrition. 4. Veganism.
5. Vegan cooking. I. Title.
RA781.B699 2015   613.7   C2015-906120-2
eBook ISBN 978-0-14-319810-9

American Library of Congress Cataloging in Publication data available

www.penguinrandomhouse.ca

CONTENTS

FOREWORD

by Venus Williams

Fitness has always been a huge part of my life. I started playing tennis at the age of four, and I recall that most of my childhood was spent playing tennis. I also spent many hours cross-training, running track, and playing other sports. This was all in the pursuit of being the best in professional tennis. Fitness was a way of life for me.

But, like anyone, I've been through ups and downs in my career, and in health in general. In 2011, I was diagnosed with Sjögren's syndrome, an autoimmune disease that can be very debilitating. Symptoms such as overwhelming fatigue consumed me, and sore and inflamed joints made it hard for me to even grip my racket. I also had terrible cravings for refined sugar, and it was getting the best of me. I gained 22 pounds. It was an extremely hard time for me, and certainly the lowest point in my career. But it taught me something: *It's not so much what happens to you that defines who you are, but rather how you deal with it.*

Getting off the sugar that I was literally chemically addicted to, and coming back from the debilitating effects of Sjögren's syndrome, taught me the meaning of true character and instilled a newfound belief in myself, which certainly made me a stronger person. There have been times when I've had to reassess my approach and come up with a new plan, especially when I felt as though the original one was not taking me in the direction I needed to go. You can't just show up on the scene thinking you are going to be on top if you haven't prepared yourself. Whatever it is you want to achieve, go about doing it by setting goals and working toward them. Don't be afraid of the hard work; in fact, the best and most memorable part of achieving success is the journey along the way!

What I appreciate about *Thrive Fitness* is that it's aimed at helping you truly get the best out of yourself. In a simple and practical manner, Brendan clearly explains the logic that went into each phase of the program's development. He holds your hand, guiding you through every aspect of fitness and nutrition. Whether you're a world-class athlete or just getting started, there's insight to be gained and progress to be made. As Brendan says, "As close as you can get to perfection is constant improvement." I truly believe this and have lived with this philosophy my entire life; I always strive to be better. And, unlike most other programs, Thrive Fitness doesn't just focus on the physical. Brendan takes a holistic approach and considers all aspects of what it really means to grow and progress into a completely fit person—from right brain stimulation for creative thought enhancement, to learning new movements in order to reduce the risk of neurological disease later in life, to a complete training and eating plan that guides you through proven ways to naturally reduce cortisol levels and produce HGH.

Fitness is not just to be enjoyed on the court, around the track, or in the gym. It's so much more than that. Once you become fit, you will have what Brendan calls "fitness capital," which will make any project you attempt easier to be successful at. Fitness capital will enable you to sleep more deeply, and therefore less will be required; it will bestow you with energy that will not need to be replenished with sugar and coffee; and it will enable you to think more clearly and be more creative, therefore turning your fitness gains into real-world success.

In 2007, I started an athletic clothing company called EleVen by Venus, and this, along with other entrepreneurial ventures, on top of being a pro tennis player, has kept me very busy. Anyone who has started a business knows exactly what I'm talking about. But, since my mental and physical fitness are a priority, I was able to achieve what many simply didn't believe could be done: simultaneously being an entrepreneur and a pro athlete. And this is not because I have some kind of innate advantage; it's simply because I capitalized on my holistic fitness to get the most out of myself.

In my tennis career the wins that I remember the most, and that have been the most rewarding, have been the ones that I have had to work the hardest for. When I was making my comeback after I was diagnosed, qualifying for the Olympics was everything for me, and I did everything I had to do to get there. Those wins make me the most proud, and those are the ones that build the most character.

Go ahead and put in the work, never set limits, and open your mind to the possibilities—they are endless. The acquisition of fitness is simply the beginning; the achievements that you will accomplish are the true benefits of holistic fitness, and that's the Thrive way!

To your success,
Venus Williams

PREFACE TO THE SECOND EDITION

Since the publication of the first edition of this book back in 2009, we've seen progress in the strides for overall health and wellness in North America. According to the American Heart Association, deaths and cardiovascular disease declined from 910,000 in 2009 to 787,000 in 2011. The economy has picked up, and, generally speaking, more people say they have an interest in where their food comes from and recognize that they can take control of their health by simply eating better and following a purposeful workout program. The relationship between food, exercise, and quality of life is better understood than ever before.

Progress is certainly nice to see; however, we still have a lot of work to do. I'm pleased to put forth this second edition of *Thrive Fitness*. Since its first publication in 2009, I've personally made significant developments, specifically to training structure and efficiency. The last few years have been a powerful learning experience for me, as I transitioned from simply an endurance athlete into a more rounded, complete athlete. I feel strongly about getting this revised and enhanced version out into the world to share what I've learned—especially as it relates to the workout program itself. I've completely reworked the program to be more dynamic, resulting in gains achieved in less time. And, unlike in the first edition, this program can be performed without any gym equipment (a basic inflatable exercise ball, a weighted ball, and push-up stands are suggested but not required), and it can now be done entirely at home, or even while traveling and staying in a basic hotel room. With this enhanced version, the absolute least amount of time and energy needs to be spent to realize the greatest fitness return. Of course, the cornerstone remains a holistic approach, with a focus not simply on strength gains and diminished body fat percentage, but rather on all that encompasses complete fitness: lasting energy, rejuvenating sleep, mental clarity, enhanced creativity, and a reduced risk of developing Alzheimer's and cardiovascular disease. Strong, lean, functional muscles and a low body fat percentage will result, but there is so much more to be gained.

A notable difference in this approach compared with many others is that this is one of synergy, not one of balance. Of course, it's common for people to suggest that we ought to strive for "balance," stating that, for good health, one must lead a balanced life that includes work and recreation. I see it differently. Balance is compromise; for one aspect to be enhanced (go up), the other must be taken from (come down), just like a scale. I don't suggest we find balance, but rather follow a complementary program.

I'm sure you've heard people say that they don't have time to work out. It's a common statement. Yet I honestly believe that I don't have time *not* to work out. I've found that the hour or so I spend training in the morning far offsets the time it consumed. The first return comes immediately in the form of endorphins that enhance drive and focus and cause a feeling of general well-being. Later in the day, a greater level of clarity, sharpness, and creativity is the result. There's no balance there—simply a purposeful, integrated holistic program that works synergistically with life. That's the Thrive Fitness program.

INTRODUCTION

For me, fitness wasn't an option. In ninth grade, I had decided that I wanted to be a professional athlete, so I had to be fit. Starting out as a track runner, it didn't take long before my strengths and weaknesses revealed themselves. Apparently, I had very little natural speed. So I figured that perhaps I would fare better in endurance sports. But I didn't. My ability to run for a long time without fatigue setting in wasn't particularly impressive either. With no speed and little endurance, I would either have to rethink my career goals or find out how to dramatically improve.

Despite these shortcomings, I genuinely enjoyed running. Each morning before school, I would run around the track for 10 minutes. Even in that brief amount of time, I began to appreciate some of running's many attributes. It served as a "mental time-out"—little new information entered my mind, and the thoughts I already had were given a new dimension. The relaxing nature of running became a form of escapism. And I was improving. Each week I was noticeably covering more ground within 10 minutes, yet expending no extra energy.

Perhaps I wasn't overly talented as an athlete, but one of this endurance sport's greatest qualities is that talent has little bearing on who will be successful. To be a great sprinter, for example, your muscles must be predominantly made up of fast-twitch fibers—a trait determined by genetics. For endurance pursuits, you just have to do your chosen sport over and over. The training effect will take hold and performance will improve. Without fail, slowly and methodically chipping away will forge the lean, efficient muscularity and cardiovascular system of a high-level athlete. The greatest determining factor for success is simply "putting in the miles." And since I enjoyed doing that, the odds shifted in my favor.

The more I ran, the more it became obvious that I actually did have a talent of sorts—the ability to recognize that I was average at best and would have to work harder and smarter than others to achieve any level of success. I accepted that I would have to put in thousands of hours of endurance training to have a chance to race professionally.

And it worked. I turned my "talent" into a career. Graduating from high school in 1993, I began my professional Ironman triathlon career in 1998. Having raced pro for seven years, in the autumn of 2003 I was hit by a car while cycling. Though I wasn't injured badly, I wasn't able to race the following year. Having been completely immersed in full-time training and racing since high school, the only people I kept company with were like-minded high-level endurance athletes, so, to me, we were "normal." As I began to meet people outside of my athletes-only circle of friends, I started to realize how fortunate I was to be highly fit. I got a glimpse of its value in a real-world setting and started to appreciate what higher-level fitness could offer in terms of high-quality living. I noticed significant differences from those who were of average or below-average fitness: I had no cravings for sugary, starchy foods or caffeine-containing drinks. I didn't require much sleep—seven hours a night was plenty—since I slept deeply and woke up feeling completely revitalized and ready to go. My energy level was always high with-

out reliance on stimulants. My thoughts were clear from early morning to late at night. I was viewed as a bit of an oddity by my new circle of friends.

Once you become fit, you accumulate what I call "fitness capital." While fitness alone offers many benefits, its greatest attribute is the platform it provides on which to build peak performance in any facet of life. It's what you do with your fitness that's most valuable. Capitalizing on an abundance of energy, mental clarity, and the necessary drive to maintain fitness will lead to significant life-improving results. Fitness will improve the odds of success in your chosen pursuit. I now view fitness as the development of something much bigger, something far more important than athletic success.

Nutrition has also proved to be an integral part of my athletic program when training full-time, and I truly appreciate the synergy between high-quality whole food consumption and exercise. Since training breaks down muscle tissue and food rebuilds it, exercise and nutrition were the two chief elements of my successful bid to become a professional athlete. Having adopted a completely plant-based diet at the age of 15, I had refined its subtleties over the years to synergistically complement my training for quick and lasting results.

Having had some success with my first book, *The Thrive Diet* (Penguin Canada, 2007), I developed a small following. Initially, my approach attracted only athletes who ate a plant-based diet. As interest spread, however, my diet program eventually garnered mainstream appeal. Why, I'm not exactly sure, but I would guess it had to do with the fact that our health as a society was on a steady decline, and conventional medicine was not providing all the answers. The general public was gradually beginning to appreciate that the combination of regular exercise and sound nutrition was a form of preventative medicine significantly bolstering quality of life and preventing the need for symptom-treating drugs later in life. I also believe that the increased focus on environmental issues and bids for preservation created a shift in consciousness and therefore interest. The understanding that we are dependent on our food-producing earth for sustenance was a new concept to some, but became relevant to all.

In the spring of 2006, on behalf of the Physicians Committee for Responsible Medicine (PCRM), I was invited to speak at a congressional briefing on Capitol Hill. The plan was to present information about nutrition and its relationship to general health. Pretty simple. We needed to get the U.S. Congress to understand the parallel between what we as a society eat and the decline of our physical and mental health. Of course, since we were presenting to the government, we also needed to tie in the economy and relay how better health could translate into improved economic conditions.

Prior to the briefing, I reviewed a few statistics, in particular some numbers that linked the current North American lifestyle to the sharp decline of our overall health. Quite honestly, the magnitude of the problem was shocking. (I provide more detail in Chapter 1). To my astonishment, however, the solution was almost as shocking in its simplicity. We didn't need high-end technology, outlandishly expensive super-drugs, or risky procedures. The obesity, the rapidly declining standard of life, and the premature deaths—not to mention the money spent on symptom-treating drugs and the skyrocketing medical costs—could be eliminated by two things: regular physical activity and sound nutrition. That was it. But if the solution was so simple, why were we in this predicament? And, more importantly, how could we get out of it?

That was when I decided to write this book. If there were two things I knew about, it was exercise and good nutrition. Having had a seven-year career as a professional Ironman triathlete whose success hinged on the quality of food eaten, I was confident I could make a contribution. Over the years, I had gathered the knowledge to apply sound physical training and nutrition to enable me to steadily improve year after year and remain competitive.

It became clear to me that many people don't understand what constitutes good nutrition, and even if they do, they are unable to integrate it into the (now-standard) hectic, time-starved life that most of us lead. And what about exercise? Most of us simply don't feel there's enough time in the day to fit it in.

> we don't have to rely
> on others; we can take
> charge of our future

I wanted to create a "real world" program. Having experienced the benefits firsthand while racing full-time, I appreciated what I had gained. But,

clearly, exercising several hours a day is not practical for most people—and, as I found later, it's not necessary either. I set out to create a functional lifestyle that fit our modern schedules.

As I began developing and writing *Thrive Fitness*, my initial idea morphed into a more comprehensive, far-reaching plan than I had originally intended. It was no longer just a program to improve the physical body. Of course, it helps to reduce body fat, build lean, functional muscles, significantly reduce the risk of cardiovascular disease, and boost mental prowess, but there is more. While it is common for exercise programs to end once fitness is obtained, or to switch into maintenance mode, Thrive Fitness is a way of life. With this in mind, I developed a web series that is complementary to this way of living, called Thrive Forward. It consists of 40-plus videos, downloadable recipes, and customizable meal plans. And it's all free at www .thriveforward.com.

WHAT HAPPENED TO OUR HEALTH?

The best way to predict your future is to create it

— Abraham Lincoln

THE DECLINE OF OUR WELL-BEING

Western society is in a state of health never seen in history. We are fatter, less productive, and at a higher risk for developing disease, early osteoporosis, and clinical depression than ever before. Why? We eat too much of the wrong types of food, not enough of the right types, and we are not sufficiently physically active.

Somewhere along the line, the modern world, with its hectic schedules, has pulled the rug out from under us. We have lost sight of our basic needs. We have stopped taking care of ourselves. And that's become a problem—a big problem. In fact, it's developed into an epidemic and one of the greatest challenges of our time. True, we are living longer, but our quality of life is questionable as our general health is at an all-time low.

According to the American Heart Association, 787,000 Americans die each year due to cardiovascular disease. (The Heart and Stroke Foundation reports more than 69,500 Canadian deaths annually from cardiovascular disease.) That's the death-toll equivalent of a 9/11 every 33 hours. Although cardiovascular disease is almost completely preventable by means of a healthy diet and regular exercise, we allow the death toll to mount rapidly and—to make matters worse—we commonly justify it. Sadly, many people rationalize a sharp decline in health as a natural part of aging. But to have high blood pressure, elevated cholesterol, an obese body, and joints so inflamed you have trouble getting out of a chair—all at the age of 40—is not natural. Unfortunately, however, it is becoming average, even normal.

We have chosen to define the word *health* as, simply, the absence of disease. That's it. "Not being sick" is good enough. To me, it seems we have set an

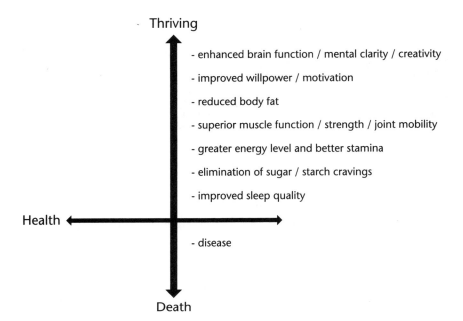

Thriving

- enhanced brain function / mental clarity / creativity

- improved willpower / motivation

- reduced body fat

- superior muscle function / strength / joint mobility

- greater energy level and better stamina

- elimination of sugar / starch cravings

- improved sleep quality

Health

- disease

Death

awfully low standard. Existing in a disease-free state is the start, but by no means the pinnacle, of health. We can have so much more. And I know that if you're reading this book, that's what you want out of life.

How can we achieve more than simply "not being sick"? As mentioned in the Introduction, the solution is considerably easier than you might expect, given the scale and duration of this epidemic. If we simply focus on ourselves— if we pour resources into ourselves, take care of ourselves—we can fix the problem.

When you board an airplane and are seated, the cabin crew reviews the safety procedures. No matter what airline you fly with, there's always a statement to the effect that, should the cabin pressure drop, oxygen masks will fall from the ceiling. The crew instructs you to put on and secure your own mask before assisting others. Excellent advice. You're of no use to anyone else if you're not breathing. To effectively help others, you must first help yourself. You need to be selfish in the true sense of the word. Taking this idea a step further, our ability to help others and bring about positive change in the world will be far greater and considerably more effective if we are in top form. To truly make a difference, our well-being is not a nicety, it's essential.

Of course, today we think it is an insult to be referred to as selfish. But should we? I suggest that we need to cultivate several forms of selfishness for our self-development, self-improvement, and self-revitalization if we are to raise our quality of living and that of those around us.

To achieve peak health and enjoy all its benefits, each of us needs to make time on a regular basis to focus on self-development. By spending as little as 45 minutes three times a week to significantly reduce our risk of all types of disease, improve sleep quality, eliminate junk food cravings, boost energy, lose body fat, and gain lean, functional muscles that move with grace and ease is, in my estimation, time well spent.

If we all focused on our own well-being, one of the greatest crises of our time would be abolished. As a society, we would no longer be susceptible to that laundry list of ailments now considered "normal." While I realize that it is unrealistic for everyone to take part, those who do will make a considerable difference. They will experience measured and clearly defined advances in both physical and mental health and thus improve their standard of living: higher quality of sleep, reduced or eliminated cravings for sugary foods, even and ever-present calm energy, and the ability to think clearly. Although these gains are significant in themselves, what we can achieve because of them is even more valuable.

The ability to work harder, sleep less, and generally be more productive can serve as a platform for building success in all aspects of our lives.

taking time to improve ourselves benefits everyone around us

THE OBESITY EPIDEMIC

In addition to our sharply declining cardiovascular health, North Americans are in the middle of an obesity epidemic, according to press releases from the U.S. Centers for Disease Control and Prevention (CDC).

This first became obvious to me during a book tour a few years ago. I was speaking to several groups in and around Chicago and was scheduled to continue to Washington, D.C., for a series of lectures. I didn't find out until I was in Illinois that one of my talks in Washington would be the dinner keynote address at the Humane Society of the United States' annual conference. I realized that I hadn't packed formal-enough clothing. Since I was staying in downtown Chicago, right near Michigan Avenue—the shopping mecca of the city—I figured I would simply walk into any men's clothing store, buy a suit jacket, and be on my way.

It wasn't that simple. After visiting no fewer than six stores and trying on a dozen jackets, I discovered that although there were many jackets on offer, there wasn't one that even came close to fitting me. Several jackets were long enough but were clearly cut to fit a person with considerable weight around the midsection. The jackets hung off of me as though I were a scarecrow. I have a lean, 170-pound frame and am about six feet, one inch tall. I had never seen that as a problem—until that day.

Getting frustrated, I asked a salesperson why it was so difficult to find a suit jacket that fit. After briefly looking me up and down, he replied, "It's 'cause we're all getting fatter." Simple answer. And the correct one, as I would later learn. He then said, "Let me measure you." Within about 20 seconds he had done the necessary measurements. "You're a 38 tall. We haven't carried those since the mid-1990s."

I later discovered that in order to keep up with the escalating girth of consumers, clothing manufacturers increase the size of their garments (the actual amount of fabric) without changing the size label. Or they simply change the labels. What was labeled as S 10 years ago is now labeled as XS, even though the actual garment size has remained the same. Clothing manufacturers know this helps people feel better about their escalating weight, but it does nothing to encourage them to do anything about it.

unhealthy weight gain has become the new standard

In the early 1990s, the CDC reported that being overweight or obese (defined as being 30 pounds or more above Body Mass Index, or BMI) was the underlying cause of 300,000 deaths a year in the United States. By 2000, that number had jumped to 400,000—a 33 percent increase. With a population of about 280 million, that is a significant proportion. It means that in 2000, just over 14 percent of the adult population of the United States died from complications of a completely preventable ailment—an ailment that is not at all mysterious and can be eradicated if we choose to do so. Yet its rate continues to grow.

But those who died weren't the only ones who carried around too much weight. In the early 1990s, more than half of the U.S. adult population—56 percent—was overweight or obese. That's 139 million people. A similar CDC survey conducted between 1999 and 2002 showed that that number had now increased by 43 million (the total population also grew by almost 33 million), to 65 percent. It is clear that obesity not only has a firm foothold in the United States, it is strengthening its grip.

If the incidence of obesity continues to climb, by 2019, obesity will overtake cardiovascular disease as the number-one cause of preventable death in America.

But what about Canadians? Do we fare any better? A little—but not as much as you might expect. The number of overweight and obese Canadians has also increased swiftly over the past few decades. Results from the Canadian Community Health Survey indicate that 47 percent of Canadian adults were overweight or obese in 2000–2001. That figure had risen by less than 1 percent by 2004. But a significant rise was reported the following year, indicating that 59 percent of Canadian adults were now overweight or obese. While Canadians still trail Americans in their percentage of overweight and obese citizens, they are closing in. The rate at which Canadians are becoming overweight and obese is, in fact, greater than that of Americans. This will likely come as a surprise to most Canadians. And while we may speculate about the reasons, researchers have not yet figured out why.

In the early part of the previous century, being overweight was a sign of wealth and, as such, a status symbol. Those who were able to afford excessive amounts of food wanted the world to see that they made enough money to over-eat. Fortunately, times have changed, and today people showcase their wealth in less health-damaging ways. Now, however, the other end of the income spectrum is most commonly overweight or obese. According to studies conducted by the Journal of the American Medical Association, low-income individuals and families are more likely to be overweight than those earning middle and high incomes. Of course this is a generalization, but that's how these kinds of studies work.

As you might expect, low-quality diet is one of the main reasons for the increase in obesity among the poor. Many processed and highly refined foods (or what, in some cases, are more properly referred to as edible foodlike substances) are cheaper than whole, fresh, and natural options. People with less money are more likely to buy the cheaper foods.

This is problematic for two reasons. First, highly processed and refined foods generally have little to no nutritional value. Therefore, you have to consume considerably more food to satisfy the body's need for nutrients. Only when the body has the nutrients it requires does it switch off its hunger signal. The negative short-term effect is that more food will be consumed, which leads quickly to weight gain. The digestion of this additional, low-nutrient food robs the body of energy without providing much energy in return. The result is that the person feels less full and has to spend more money to buy more food to stay satiated. If that person were to gradually switch over to a diet composed of more expensive whole foods, he or she would no longer be in a constant state of hunger and therefore would naturally choose to consume less. The financial savings gained from buying cheap processed foods quickly evaporate.

Second, the consumption of these processed foods contributes to long-term health risks. If a person has relied on processed foods to reconstruct the body day in and day out for decades, that body will falter later in life. Disease of some form will almost certainly be the result. Type II diabetes, arthritis, osteoporosis, and the many offshoots of cardiovascular disease are the most common to develop. The drugs needed to treat these ailments frequently cost several thousand dollars per month. And that's just to alleviate the symptoms; the underlying disease continues to progress. Admittedly, there are rare cases when drugs can eradicate the disease; however, what caused the disease in the first place has not been addressed, and therefore it may return.

> in the long term, eating
> nutrient-rich food costs
> less money

To put it simply, replacing refined, processed foods with natural, whole foods is a form of health insurance. You will stack the odds in your favor and save money in the long run. In the short term, you will have more energy and greater mental clarity, both of which can significantly improve productivity. Some people may choose to put a dollar value on that.

OVERFED YET UNDERNOURISHED

What was an impossible paradox only 50 years ago is now a strange reality: People who are overweight or obese in our society can, and likely will, show signs of malnutrition. Blood test studies of overweight and obese patients consistently show low levels of several vitamins and minerals as well as overall poor blood quality.

It wasn't long ago that the more a person ate, the more nourished he or she became. But not anymore. With refined foods representing the base of the North American diet, food consumption is no longer synonymous with nourishment. The greater the amount of processed food a person consumes, the greater the chance that person will become malnourished. Most refined foods do not contain the nutrients we need for good health. In fact, refined foods can actually deplete the body of the nutrients it currently has. Calcium levels, for example, will decline when refined, acid-forming foods are consumed as a staple in place of whole foods. (I explain this in detail beginning on page 132.) Choosing to eat highly refined foods that have only minimal amounts of nutrition, such as common frozen dinners, will result in a nutritional deficit, and in no way will improve nourishment.

As I wrote about extensively in my book *The Thrive Diet*, and as I note earlier, digesting low-quality food and edible foodlike substances requires large amounts of energy, yet the body receives little or no nutrient value in return. It's akin to doing work (stress) without being paid (a return). Digestion, which is a form of work, without the payoff of nutrients causes a stress response in your body. This response is accompanied by the production and release of cortisol, a destructive stress hormone. Once the level of cortisol becomes chronically elevated, this stress hormone wreaks havoc.

food no longer has the nutrition it once had

Elevated cortisol levels inhibit the body's ability to slip into the deep phase of sleep during which cellular regeneration and overall revitalization take place. Most people never experience this deep sleep. The result: They wake up tired, craving coffee and sugary foods. When they consume those refined, sugary, and caffeine-containing foods or bever-

ages, their adrenal glands are stimulated and energy is generated. But it doesn't last long. Adrenal stimulation results in quick yet fleeting energy that is always followed by fatigue. If this cycle of adrenal fatigue is allowed to continue and become a regular part of life—as it does for most of the North American population—compounded adrenal exhaustion ensues.

How many times have you said, "If I just had an extra hour in the day, I'd be able to get so much more done"? If you had lower cortisol levels—which directly equate to improved sleep quality—you would sleep more efficiently and therefore not feel the need to sleep as much, effectively creating an extra hour or so of high-quality waking time. You'd also be healthier and have the opportunity to be more productive. That is because adrenal fatigue has a host of unwelcome effects that have become chronic in our society, so much so that many of them are now considered a normal part of life.

The first signs of stress (and therefore a rise in cortisol) are commonly sleep deprivation; fatigue; mental fog; irritability; weight gain; and cravings for sugar, starch, and caffeine. These red flags play an important role. They tell us our "stress threshold" has been reached, alerting us that something is out of balance and will worsen if we don't fix it.

Unfortunately, we tend to deal with each individual symptom while ignoring the underlying cause, which is not healthy or sustainable. We use coffee and sugary foods to ward off fatigue, sleeping pills to help us sleep, and restrictive diets to assist weight loss. Over time, if we allow the underlying problems to become chronic, they can morph into serious diseases. In Chapter 2, I lay out a stress reduction plan that will allow you to eliminate a large portion of overall stress and thereby increase productivity and creativity; increase the quality of your sleep and workouts; burn fat more quickly; strengthen your immune system; decrease sugar, starch, and caffeine cravings; and significantly reduce your chances of contracting disease. I know it's a bold statement. But stress reduction through high-quality nutrition and regular exercise can deliver.

exercise, nutrition, rest, and stress reduction are intertwined

THE ECONOMIC COST

A study published in the *Washington Post* revealed that, on average, American-built automobiles cost $1,500 more than comparably equipped Japanese or European cars. The reason? Americans are in worse physical health than their Japanese and European counterparts and therefore must pay higher health insurance premiums. This addi-

tional cost is passed on to the end consumer to allow the company to maintain profitability. The United States is less competitive in the global market simply because its citizens are in a poorer state of health.

As the health of the American people declines, so, too, does the nation's economy. This is not a coincidence. More people are developing disease earlier in life than in any previous generation. Those who aren't privately insured place a tremendous burden on the taxpayer-funded healthcare system, contributing to higher taxes, a decrease in spending, a sluggish economy, and even a recession, as America is now experiencing. While there are other contributing factors here, including the sub-prime mortgage debacle and war spending, a nation made up of unhealthy people is inevitably going to become an unhealthy nation economically. A company composed of unhealthy people will never reach its full earning potential. And while the economy has strengthened over the last few years, there is still considerable room for improvement.

Large corporations are beginning to catch on. At the Googleplex in Mountain View, California, Google employees enjoy recreation facilities once the exclusive domain of high-priced resorts: a gym, two swimming pools, and a sand-volleyball court. But the Googleplex's culinary options are where it shines the brightest. With many cafeterias, the selection of food is vast. And employees can request whatever they want—whether it's on the menu or not. The cafeterias offer several balanced, plant-based options and a plethora of smoothies and raw foods.

Is Google going to this considerable up-front expense simply because they're nice people? No. They are nice, but they also understand that the improved health and happiness of their employees will improve their bottom line. And it has, consistently, since its inception in 2003. The monetary return on their investment comes in the form of employees performing at a higher level. And consider the advantages that beyond-basic health can bring to a company. Employees who are in top form have a stronger immune system and are less likely to get sick and be absent from work. Companies that don't embrace this holistic approach to well-being and productivity will not turn as great a profit and eventually will not be able to compete with the ones that do embrace it. Then they'll have to answer to their shareholders.

I can relate to this firsthand. In 2003, I met Charles Chang, who had started a natural nutrition company called Sequel Naturals the previous year. At the time, his company included him and a part-time secretary. Sequel Naturals eventually became one of my sponsors, providing me with top-of-the-line maca (MacaSure, now called Vega Maca) and premium chlorella (ChlorEssence, now called Vega Chlorella) to blend into my recovery blender drink formula. I was immediately impressed with the results, which prompted talks between Charles and me about partnering and creating a commercially available version of my blender drink formula. We turned discussion into action and a year later launched Vega in Canada and then in the United States the following year.

As Vega continued to grow, Charles hired staff and moved into a larger office. Once Vega truly developed a following, naturally the staff required to handle the demand grew steadily. Understanding the link between employee health, happiness, and performance, Charles equipped the new office with a state-of-the-art lunchroom. It is always stocked with fresh fruit, vegetables, leafy greens for salads, nuts, seeds, and, of course, Vega for making nutrient-packed smoothies. The lunchroom is open to all the employees; they are free to eat as much as they want throughout the workday.

In 2008, *Profit Magazine* listed the top 100 fastest-growing Canadian companies. With Vega soon to be four years old, Sequel Naturals (now the company is simply called Vega) was listed as the eighth fastest-growing company, with a growth of 3730 percent, and it has been on the Profit 500: Canada's Fastest-Growing Companies list from 2012 to 2015. While the health and happiness of Vega employees hasn't been the only reason for its unprecedented rate of improvement, it's undeniably been a contributing factor.

healthier people are capable of greater achievements

As I will expand on in detail in Chapter 2, the advantages of improved health and fitness are not limited to physical well-being. Improved well-being leads to greater mental clarity, greater concentration, and the ability to maintain quality of work for a longer period of time. Physical activity stimulates the subconscious, thus allowing it to do what it does best: solve problems. The subconscious has the ability to develop and bring to the conscious mind solutions to problems we had not been able to solve while actively looking for answers.

THE ENVIRONMENTAL COST

Yes, it's true: Being overweight can increase your carbon footprint. During the 1990s, the average adult American gained 10 pounds, according to the CDC. The CDC estimated that airlines had to burn an additional 350 million gallons of fuel from 1994 to 2004 just to transport their passengers' extra body weight. In addition to increasing the airlines' fuel costs by $275 million and thus creating a significant economic effect, the burning of that extra fuel released an additional 3.8 million tons of carbon dioxide into the atmosphere. That is the equivalent annual carbon dioxide emission of 13.5 million mid-size cars operating at 26 miles per gallon and traveling 155 miles per week.

Just as being overweight has a negative impact on the environment, an unhealthy environment plays a significant role in the decline of our health. Food links us to our environment. Each time we bite into food, a piece of our food-producing earth is absorbed by our bodies. Since plants are really little more than conduits for nutrients in the soil, when soil quality declines, so too does the nutritional value of our food.

The greatest contributing factor to low-nutrient food is over-farming. The land is called upon to produce more than it is capable of. And the most common reason for over-farming is the sharp rise in demand for food. But, interestingly, the demand has risen significantly to grow food to feed animals, not humans. In North America, 14 times more land is used to grow food for animals being raised for meat than to grow food for humans. And with every seven to nine pounds of food fed to a cow, for example, only one pound is returned in the form of meat. Clearly, this is inefficient. Animal agriculture is what is chiefly to blame for a decline in food quality. Though I stopped eating animal products at the age of 15 to improve health and ultimately athletic performance, not long after, I learned of the environmental benefits it offered. These findings fortified my appreciation of a plant-based diet.

While I'm pleased to see an almost worldwide genuine concern for environmental preservation, I think it's important to know that eating a plant-based diet is the single greatest thing anyone can do to personally reduce his or her environmental impact. Though installing energy-efficient light bulbs and driving a hybrid car are steps in the right direction, the adoption of a plant-based diet is a giant leap forward.

According to a 2006 Food and Agriculture Organization (FAO) of the United Nations report, livestock production has become a major threat to environmental sanctity: "Livestock are one of the most significant contributors to today's most serious environmental problems." The report concludes that livestock are responsible for 18 percent of greenhouse-gas emissions as measured in carbon dioxide equivalent. This includes 9 percent of all CO_2 emissions,

37 percent of methane, and 65 percent of nitrous oxide. These are significant numbers, to say the least. They combine to yield a total that is in fact greater than all emissions produced by transportation.

REASONS? OR EXCUSES?

According to a recent Mintel Report, the top five reasons people give for not eating well are the higher cost of healthy, whole foods; the lack of availability; confusion about what foods to eat; time constraints; and the notion that health food doesn't taste as good. I offer the following counter-arguments.

Cost: As I mentioned earlier, healthy, whole foods are actually cheaper in the long term.

Availability: Many grocery stores now have a dedicated health food aisle, and organic fruit and vegetable sections are almost the norm. The increasing number of health food stores has greatly improved the availability of high-quality food. In most urban areas, farmers' markets run eight months of the year, and healthy-meal delivery services are becoming popular.

Confusion: The information in this book and in *The Thrive Diet* is presented in a logical, clear fashion to help you make the right choices.

Time: Healthy food doesn't have to take longer to prepare. In fact, many of the Thrive recipes take less than 15 minutes. And if you need food instantly, a variety of nutritional powders, including Vega One, can serve as a premium "fast food."

Taste: Of course taste is subjective, but most people enjoy a whole food–fortified fruit smoothie. With the huge variety of ingredients available, everybody should be able to find at least a couple of recipes they truly enjoy.

Not surprisingly, with the exception of taste, people give the same reasons for not being physically active. So how do those excuses hold up?

Cost: Gym memberships are becoming more affordable—and the gym atmosphere can provide encouragement and support. But you don't need a gym membership to be physically active. Many fitness programs or activities can be performed with minimal equipment. All you need for Thrive Fitness is an inflatable exercise ball, push-up stands, and a weighted ball. This will cost less than $50 total.

Availability: Numerous fitness programs, including all the Thrive Fitness exercises, can be performed at home.

Confusion: With the information in this book, I aim to clarify how you can achieve well-being through exercise.

Time: All it takes is just 45 minutes three times a week to make significant gains.

AT A GLANCE

- North America's greatest killer—cardiovascular disease—is a disease that is nearly 100 percent preventable through sound nutrition and regular exercise.
- Taking time to focus on your own well-being will significantly improve your quality of life as well as the standard of living of those around you.
- Eating high-quality food will save you money in the long run.
- Most people in North America are overfed yet undernourished.
- The health of the people becomes the health of the nation.
- Healthier people are able to achieve more.

WHAT IS THRIVE FITNESS?

Fitness lays the foundation on which a
higher standard of living can be built

THE 4 COMPONENTS OF VITALITY

2

PROGRAM OR LIFESTYLE?

Most conventional fitness and training books focus on weight loss and its aesthetic benefits. They present a program to be completed in a set amount of time and often include before-and-after pictures. The results—toned, lean muscles and a reduction in body fat—are visually impressive and can serve to motivate people.

But Thrive Fitness encourages you to view these benefits as byproducts of your increased fitness level rather than your ultimate goal. The real benefit is what you can achieve once you have obtained fitness. A fit person can do things the non-fit person couldn't even imagine.

Thrive Fitness has no true beginning or end. Like a fitness program, it will result in linear, successive physical and mental gains—usually within 8 to 12 weeks. But those gains will be ongoing;

therefore, I prefer to view Thrive Fitness as a lifestyle.

Once you have a firm grasp of its premise, Thrive Fitness will simply become part of your life. You'll want it to. Even if your lifestyle has never included regular exercise, Thrive Fitness will help you begin a new and tremendously rewarding chapter in your life. If you are a seasoned athlete, Thrive Fitness may help you become more efficient, more focused, and able to perform at a higher level.

Initially, the physical and mental rewards will be the catalyst that makes you continue, but eventually you may also begin to enjoy the process of developing the results. In fact, the process itself contributes to many of the mental benefits of living Thrive Fitness; if you enjoy something, you are more likely to become successful at it.

There's nothing wrong with putting other areas of your life on hold and training hard to lose weight and build muscle during one 12-week period. But I believe that an ongoing, enjoyable, sustainable lifestyle that includes a fitness element is the best way to achieve your goals. You cannot reach those goals if you don't have the physical and mental fortitude to achieve them.

Thrive Fitness lays the foundation for peak mental and physical health and vitality. Once you are not just healthy but thriving, everything you do in life will be easier—whatever your goals and wherever you choose to focus your newfound energy, drive, and ambition.

The Thrive Fitness program has four components of vitality. There are two core elements—high-return exercise and high net-gain nutrition—supported by two less appreciated factors that, in many cases, are the glue holding the core together—efficient sleep and uncomplementary stress reduction.

High-Return Exercise

Physical exercise is really nothing more than breaking down body tissue—thus encouraging the body to grow back stronger than it was. High-return exercise is only performing an exercise when a solid return on your energy investment is ensured; therefore, it is a core principle of Thrive Fitness. When combined with low-energy output, high-return exercise will help quickly build muscular strength that will result in greater efficiency and therefore will have a major impact on all aspects of life—from greater energy levels, reduced body fat, and better mental clarity to reduced risk of disease.

High Net-Gain Nutrition

Based on my Thrive philosophy (outlined in *The Thrive Diet*), this component outlines why easily digestible, nutrient-dense whole foods are the cornerstone of an effective nutrition plan. The premise is simple: stress reduction through better nutrition. Eating more high net-gain foods maximizes efficient digestion and assimilation of nutrients and eliminates excess work for the body. As a large amount of nutritional stress is relieved, symptoms such as general fatigue and sugar and starch cravings will disappear.

Efficient Sleep

This component describes how high-quality sleep, or deep sleep, expedites the benefits of an exercise and nutrition program. The result of exercise—broken-down cells—combined with the building blocks provided by high net-gain nutrition—to grow back stronger cells—go to work in this phase of sleep. To sleep deeply is to sleep efficiently.

Better-rested people have more energy and aren't reliant upon stimulants such as sugar or caffeine to get it.

Uncomplementary Stress Reduction

While nutritional stress, and therefore a large part of overall stress, can be attributed to poor diet, there are several lifestyle situations that also cause stress responses. Reducing the amount of work you perform will, in most cases, reduce stress. But what about productivity? How does one reduce stress while maintaining a productive life? While the goal of general stress reduction is a good one, we must be mindful to focus our efforts on eliminating uncomplementary stress while maintaining complementary and production stress. In *The Thrive Diet*, I explain each stress and its origins in great detail. And more importantly, I outline how to selectively reduce unbeneficial types of stress while cultivating activities that, although stress producing, will benefit our lives and help us achieve our goals.

In addition, consistently doing things that you don't enjoy is a major contributing factor to stress. The way you perceive what you're doing is of utmost importance. I explain the value of perception, its role on stress, and how to ensure your lifestyle is structured in a way that will allow for complementary enjoyment.

As you will discover, each of these four components is dependent on the others, as shown on the next page.

HIGH-RETURN EXERCISE

The Breakthrough

In 1990, when I first began training with the ambition of becoming a premier endurance athlete, I performed countless hours of slow- to moderate-paced, easy training: an hour and a half in the pool, an hour at the gym, between four and six hours of cycling, and about an hour and a quarter of running. This training took the better part of the day to complete and left me exhausted by sundown. But my times gradually and steadily improved: Each year I placed higher.

> a greater level of fitness makes achieving any goal easier

The patient approach I had taken was paying off. But it was a lot of work, and, to make matters worse, I had to keep on increasing the distance and therefore the time I spent training to maintain my steady improvement. Food preparation, food consumption, the training itself, and the post-training stretching took up so much of my time that the days evaporated at an alarming rate. And all these activities represented a significant energy draw. By the time I'd completed

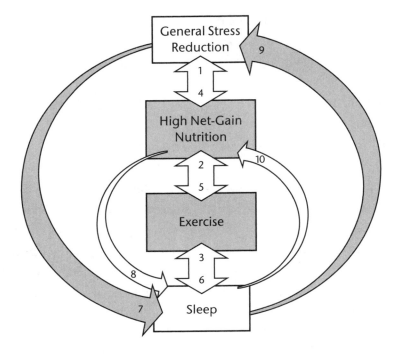

1. High net-gain nutrition reduces overall stress.
2. Exercise breaks down muscle tissue cells and therefore allows good nutrition to re-build cells.
3. Better rest leads to more energy and hence better quality exercise.
4. Reduced stress leads to fewer junk food cravings.
5. Better nutrition creates a stronger body and hence fuels better exercise performance.
6. Moderate exercise improves sleep quality.
7. Reduced stress leads to lower cortisol levels and hence improved sleep quality.
8. High net-gain nutrition reduces overall stress and therefore improves sleep quality.
9. High-quality sleep reduces cortisol levels and overall stress.
10. Better quality sleep leads to fewer junk food cravings.

the last workout of the day, I would be fatigued to the point of not being able to do anything but slump in a chair. And since my thoughts had been wandering the whole day during training, by the evening I just wanted a distraction to stop myself from thinking. Watching TV was all I could handle.

Eventually, I was dedicating about 10 hours a day to training. Since I was no longer able to add time to my training, my fitness level reached a plateau. The energy I was putting in simply wasn't producing the returns it once did. Had I reached my potential?

I spoke with other high-level athletes and found that most of them accepted very small incremental improvements relative to their level of energy expenditure. "That's just the way it is" was the attitude. The fitter an athlete becomes, the smaller the gains.

As with any pursuit, the more proficient one becomes, the smaller the improvements become. For example, if a world-class speaker were to sign up for a class at a community college called "Speaking 101: How to Overcome Your Fear of Public Speaking," he or she would clearly be wasting time and energy.

The same holds true for physical training. If an extremely out-of-shape, sedentary person, for example, were to begin performing five minutes of jumping jacks three times a week, that person's fitness level would improve. However, if a highly trained cyclist were to incorporate five minutes of jumping jacks into his or her routine three times a week, it would not challenge the body at all. The cyclist's fitness level is already so high that it cannot be improved by such an easy, non-specific exercise.

> spending time and energy wisely is vital for continual improvement

I was experiencing this phenomenon firsthand. And I wasn't happy about it. But what was the solution? I racked my brain, reviewing my training and nutrition. And then it dawned on me. Something I had never even considered before. Not realizing it, I had become narrow-minded and complacent in my training approach. As an endurance athlete, I trained for endurance the only way I knew how: by performing copious amounts of long, low-intensity training. As long as I was improving, I remained satisfied. But with satisfaction came complacency. The training was working, but was I getting the best return on my energy and time investment? Energy is the most common expenditure that we make on a regular basis. But how often do we consider the return on our investment and whether a particular activity is a sensible way to spend our precious resource?

Return on Investment

Many people cite low energy as one of their top problems, yet they spend their energy on activities that offer little or no return. They had energy to begin with; they simply made a bad investment choice. Spending energy to digest refined, processed food, for instance, is not a wise investment when the alternative is clear (I'll go into detail about this on page 41). We all have a finite amount of energy. And conserving our energy is more effective than trying to obtain more. If you don't have much money, for example, you would be wise to stop spending what little you have on nonessential items. Buying a new car every couple of years, fancy clothing, and household goods can only lead to one thing: less money. But if you spend what little money you have on an item that will increase in value and give you back more money than you put into it, you would be making a good investment. The same is true for exercise. Spending more energy to exercise a greater amount is not necessarily a wise investment. In fact, in many cases, less is better. But in all cases, some exercise is essential.

Most of the time, you invest time, effort, and energy exercising, and the return is a healthier, more robust you.

Pretty straightforward. So when is exercise not a good investment? When do you risk expending more energy than you are likely to gain back? There is no simple answer. As the graph below shows, if the energy investment remains constant, the return decreases during each successive training section.

Since we all have busy lives and many opportunities to spend our energy, we must decide at what point would we rather spend our energy elsewhere or, alternatively, invest it more wisely to yield a better return. Is it possible to change the principal of your investment to gain a larger payback?

Absolutely yes. Sensible, well-calculated energy expenditure to gain maximum returns is one of the core components of Thrive Fitness. For me, the pursuit of a better investment would lead to the creation of Thrive Fitness.

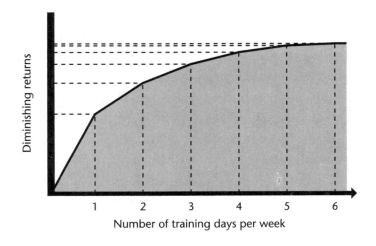

Diminishing returns

Number of training days per week

*for optimal fitness gain,
only make investments that
yield a worthy return*

More Effective Training

I figured that if I took a closer, more scientific look at what was actually happening when I was training, a better way of exercising might present itself. While I knew that countless factors come together to compose a successful endurance athlete, the two prime elements are cardiovascular fitness and muscular strength. If both these elements are strong and performing at an equal rate, performance will be solid.

In order to break through the plateau I had settled at, I needed to figure out my next steps. So I made a trip to the sports performance laboratory in Vancouver, where I was put through my paces to see how I measured up.

I ran on a treadmill while my vitals were monitored on a computer. A breathing apparatus was inserted into my mouth, and a clip was put on my nose to prevent any air leaving or entering through my nose. That way, all the air that entered and exited my system could be monitored and measured. Every few minutes, the oxygen saturation of my blood was measured. The protocol was for me to run at a steadily increasing pace until the exhaustion became more than I could bear. Since the pace of the treadmill was being increased every two minutes, it was estimated that I'd have to stop running at about 20 minutes. I made it to about the 22-minute mark, but that was it, the intensity had ramped up to a point that I was unable to take in enough oxygen to supply the requirements of my muscles. I had been "maxed out."

The outcome was fascinating. It shed light on what I had overlooked for years in my training. The test indicated that my heart was in good shape. No surprise there. It was described as "pumping blood throughout my body in a strong and deliberate fashion." My tireless hours of aerobic training had built a strong heart.

However, my muscular system did not fare as well. My legs showed signs of fatigue considerably earlier in the test than did my heart. Performance in an endurance sport, as with many things, is only as good as the weakest link. And my muscles were my weak link. But how could that be? I spent hours every day swimming, cycling, and running, all of which require thousands of muscle contractions. Why had my muscles not made the gains in endurance that I expected from all that relentless endurance training? And, more to the point, what could I do about it? I certainly couldn't train any more. I would have to train smarter.

increased muscular strength reduces the strain placed on the heart

I needed to rework my strategy. This was my problem: Aside from the heart and the rest of the cardiovascular system, the muscles, primarily those of the legs, need to be in top form to obtain peak performance. With each muscle contraction, energy is expended. The amount of energy needed to cause a muscle to contract is based on two main factors: the size of the muscle and, more importantly, the efficacy of the muscle. The fitter the muscle, the less energy the body needs to cause it to contract. That's important. An endurance athlete gains a large benefit when energy can be conserved with each muscle contraction. The endurance cyclist, for example, will contract his or her leg muscles 180 times per minute when cycling at an average cadence of 90 rotations per minute. That equates to 10,800 contractions per hour of the largest muscle group in the body—the gluteus maximus, quadriceps, hamstrings, and to a lesser degree the gastrocnemius muscles. Even a modest savings in energy expenditure to perform a muscle contraction will

yield significant energy conservation. Of course, when you don't spend energy, you still have it. Improving muscle efficiency is a phenomenal energy booster.

That was it. I needed to get stronger to improve my endurance. I began lifting weights, with the expectation of developing stronger muscles. After a few weeks I noticed I was making progress. I looked stronger—well, bigger anyway. I had gained about eight pounds. But this extra strength didn't seem to be doing me any good. My running and cycling times actually got slower. What was happening? As I discovered, I was getting modestly stronger, yet since my weight was also increasing, my strength-to-weight ratio was actually declining. For an endurance athlete, that's a red flag. Endurance athletes need to be strong yet remain light, so that it takes less energy for their muscles to move. The energy that is saved can be used to improve endurance and ultimately performance.

stronger muscles reduce overall stress that the body must endure

So why was the weight training not working for me? As I discovered, most weight training programs are built on one variation or another of a traditional bodybuilding philosophy. Bodybuilders are unique athletes. While it may seem odd, strength is not an important component of their sport, and muscle functionality, efficiency, fluidity, and strength-to-weight ratio play no part. Rather, the goal of bodybuilding is to develop large, thick muscle mass with symmetry and definition. The winner is assessed on appearance only.

In the 1970s, modern bodybuilding rose to mainstream popularity and began the fitness craze that would span the decade and spill over into the 1980s. It is thought that the now-legendary documentary *Pumping Iron*—shot primarily at Gold's Gym in Venice Beach, California ("the mecca of bodybuilding"), and chronicling a brash 28-year-old Arnold Schwarzenegger's bid to win a sixth consecutive Mr. Olympia bodybuilding title in 1975—kick-started the imagination of American people who aspired to become fit, if only in appearance. Bodybuilding is undeniably a sport—but it should not be considered synonymous with strength training. In fact, many consider bodybuilding to be a form of performance art. It's beautiful to some, but by no means is bodybuilding pursued for the sake of practicality, functionality, or health.

To propel my endurance to the next level, I needed a program that would build strength without increasing bulk. But because of all the endurance training I still needed to perform for my cardiovascular fitness, I wanted a strength training program that required little time or energy investment. And while I enjoy going to the gym, I wanted the option, if pressed for time, to be able to perform the program at home with limited equipment. These were tall orders.

I began experimenting with higher-intensity strength training. Within a short time, results began to reveal themselves. This was exciting. Not since the early days had I experienced such improvement in endurance in such a short time frame and after only a small energy expenditure. As I refined the program and allowed it to organically evolve over the years based on carefully gauging my performance in a logbook, I arrived at a system that was remarkably solid. It yielded top returns on energy, time, and effort.

bigger muscles don't necessarily mean stronger muscles

In fact, this system was so effective at increasing strength with minimal time and effort that I was able to significantly cut back on the amount of endurance training I performed. I went from training 10 hours a day to 3—a 70 percent drop. Even more notably, my endurance did not level off (as I had feared it might); it actually improved. I was astounded. By creating peak muscular strength while exerting only small amounts of energy, I had broken through to the upper echelons. And I had so much more time and energy for other activities. The extra energy simply came from better investment choices. I wasn't spending nearly as much, and as a result I had more. Plus, since I was no longer logging monstrous training miles, the chances of reaching my stress threshold—and possibly overtraining—greatly diminished.

This amazing realization changed the way I thought about training and building fitness. I maintained the premise of my new exercise plan but adapted it for the "real world." Thrive Fitness allows you to achieve peak efficacy without specific equipment and without spending copious hours of time. A tight parallel can be drawn between that of daily living and an endurance event. In fact, I don't hesitate to say that the demands of modern life are closely akin to those placed on a competitive endurance athlete. There is no choice but to keep pushing through. And I don't feel as though I'm exaggerating when I suggest that life is an endurance sport. Thrive Fitness is an exceptionally good way to improve overall efficacy and therefore fitness. In-

creased efficacy places less strain on the heart and other muscles that you rely upon daily, and as a result, you will experience a considerable increase in energy levels and a reduction in stress and its debilitating symptoms.

Strength equals efficiency. But endurance athletes aren't the only ones to benefit. Building strong, functional muscles that move with grace and ease is the cornerstone of Thrive Fitness. The less energy we exert to cause a muscle contraction, the better. Ease of movement with minimum effort is a wonderful thing. While fluidity may be the result, improved functional strength is the basis on which grace of movement can be built.

modern life is an endurance sport that requires appropriate training

With ease of movement comes a reduction of stress. Since work is simply a form of stress, the less work we can create for ourselves, the less strain we put on ourselves.

The reduction of stress leads to a reduction of cortisol levels. Lowered cortisol levels reduce the chance of developing sickness and allow the body to build lean muscle more easily, lose fat more quickly, and sleep better. Starting on page 51, I explain the value and methods of stress reduction in detail.

Spending Heartbeats Wisely

As I found out, the role of muscular strength could not be understated in my bid to become a better endurance athlete. Since stronger muscles are more efficient muscles, they are less of a draw on the heart. And that holds true not just for high-level athletic activity but also for day-to-day activity.

Consider this comparison. If your legs are weak, a higher percentage of their overall strength is needed, for example, to ascend a flight of stairs. More blood is required, causing the heart to pump faster. If, however, you are able to walk up a flight of stairs using only a fraction of your legs' strength, your climb requires less blood to be pumped throughout the body; your heart doesn't have to work as hard.

All muscles become stronger when they are used and then given time and nutrients to regenerate. The heart muscle is no exception. And the stronger the heart becomes, the more efficiently it is able to do its job of pumping blood around the body. The amount of blood that can be pumped with each beat is referred to as the heart's stroke volume. As the heart becomes stronger, so, too, does its stroke volume. The greater the stroke volume the better, since the heart will be able to pump the same volume of blood around the body while using fewer beats (that is, muscle contractions). Of course, a heartbeat uses energy. The fewer heartbeats required, the less energy expended. Once the heart gets stronger with exercise and its efficacy improves as a result, it won't need to work as hard to perform the same job. Efficacy equals energy savings. As I mentioned earlier, one of the best ways to increase the overall amount of energy you have is to limit the amount you spend on activities that offer no return. Since our hearts beat constantly, even a small savings in efficacy will translate to a significant energy gain.

> stronger muscles move
> with fluidity and embody
> greater functionality

Have you ever heard the expression—usually uttered by those who don't enjoy exercise—we only have so many heartbeats and we must spend them wisely? This belief goes back to ancient India, where yogis would focus on their breath during meditation in an effort to slow their heart rate. Conserving heartbeats was thought to prolong life; if the heart beat too much, it would wear out prematurely.

Well, there is some truth to this. It is, in fact, advantageous for us to reduce the amount of work our heart needs to perform. Since it never gets a break throughout our entire life, it can wear down. However, reducing activity to slow its beating is not the best long-term approach. While deep breathing and meditation can improve our overall health for several reasons, building a stronger, more efficient heart is the key to longevity. A stronger heart beats more efficiently and therefore does not have to beat as often.

The average at-rest heart rate for an adult who's in reasonable health is between 70 and 75 beats per minute (bpm). Performing daily activity such as walking, office work, and eating will typically increase an average person's heart rate to between 85 and 90 bpm.

Line A on the graph represents an average person in good health during a typical day. The average heart rate of 88 bpm gives a daily total of 126,720 beats.

If this same person began exercising 30 minutes a day, his or her average heart rate would be elevated to about 150 bpm for the duration of the exercise. This equates to 1,900 additional beats. But although exercise initially increases the heart rate, eventually its effect will be to bring down the total number of beats needed over the course of a day.

those with a strong, efficient
heart have more energy

Line B represents the same person with exercise incorporated into his or her daily schedule. The heart rate spikes to 150 bpm during exercise, but then it regulates for the rest of the day. After about three months of regular exercise, the average heart rate drops, as shown in the graph. When the heart gets stronger from exercise, it begins pumping more efficiently and therefore doesn't need to pump as often. The benefits are significant. The person's heart rate is down to

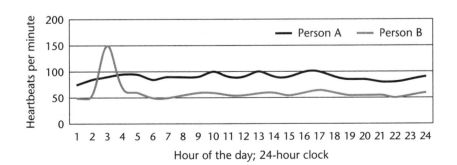

about 59 bpm, or 84,960 a day, when not exercising. That is 41,760 fewer beats every day.

Most of us spend the bulk of our day operating at a moderate heart rate. In that sense, daily life is an endurance sport. A lower average heart rate is a valuable asset for anyone, but especially for a high-performance athlete. If an athlete starts an exercise session with a lower heart rate, it will take that athlete longer to reach his or her anaerobic threshold. Anaerobic threshold, sometimes referred to as the lactate threshold, is the point at which the body can no longer remove waste products and therefore performance declines.

Another excellent way to reduce the energy requirements of your heart is to improve your maximal oxygen consumption. Abbreviated to VO_2 max, it is a measure by which aerobic fitness can be gauged. A VO_2 max test shows the maximum amount of oxygen that an individual can transport and utilize during incrementally increased exercise intensity. While it can be performed on either an exercise bike or a treadmill, the treadmill will yield the most accurate results. During the test, the speed and incline are increased until the runner is forced to stop because of fatigue. In many cases, the runner collapses from exhaustion.

AT A GLANCE

- Thrive Fitness is a lifestyle, not merely a program. Its gains go way beyond fitness.
- Better muscle tone and lower body fat are a byproduct of Thrive Fitness, rather than the ultimate goal.
- Thrive Fitness provides a high return on energy and time investment. Therefore peak fitness can be built quickly and efficiently.
- Stronger muscles move with greater ease, fluidity, and grace.
- Increased muscular strength reduces the heart's workload and therefore boosts energy.
- Increased maximal oxygen consumption (VO_2 max) can significantly improve overall health and greatly reduce the risk of heart disease. Oxygen consumption can be improved in a short amount of time and with minimal energy expenditure.

even a modest boost in VO$_2$
max will significantly improve
performance and reduce risk
of cardiovascular disease

Those with a high VO$_2$ max can use oxygen more efficiently, thus reducing strain on the body. It's not just athletes who benefit from an improved VO$_2$ max. Increased VO$_2$ max has real-world advantages that include reduced risk for cardiovascular disease, respiratory ailments, and general fatigue, as well as improved fitness and overall health. Even a modest boost in VO$_2$ max has been shown to dramatically improve cardiovascular fitness levels. On page 125 I explain how you can raise your VO$_2$ max in under 20 minutes per week.

The Non-Physical
Benefits of Exercise

As I mentioned in the Introduction, I first began running as a means to get fitter. Compared to most kids, I had begun skating and playing hockey late, at the age of 13, which put me at a disadvantage. I thought that if I were in better shape than those more experienced kids, it would level the playing field. It didn't—I was still a bad hockey player. However, while I was getting in shape for hockey, I discovered that I liked running. Eventually I stopped

playing hockey altogether, and running became my athletic focus.

As my fitness developed over the weeks and months, I no longer had to concentrate on the act of running. At a moderate pace, it had become effortless. This is the point at which everything changed for me. Because I didn't have to engage in conscious thought to be able to run, my mind would wander. Ideas I could never have imagined as belonging to me would flow every time I ran, almost as though my head were a radio receiving signals from outside. A whole other part of my brain had been accessed.

After a while, I developed the ability to come up with viable solutions to problems I had been actively thinking about and mulling over for months. After puzzling over a dilemma, actively trying to find a solution only to come up with nothing, solutions seemed to just pop into my head during a run. While I began running to improve my physical fitness, I continued running to maintain my newfound thought patterns. I don't want to suggest that I've become dependent on them, but I certainly appreciate the way in which I can tap in to creativity that I hadn't realized I had. As my fitness and running improved, so did my ability to spontaneously come up with ideas. Some weren't very good, but that was okay, since it only takes one or two sensible ideas to make a difference. I found that as the new ideas became older ideas, my brain would subconsciously sift through them while I was running and, without any active thought, separate the good from the bad.

physical exercise helps stimulate creative thought

If you've read *The Thrive Diet*, you may have noticed that I dedicated the book to Lynn, Seymour, and Stanley. Each is a large park in the Vancouver area. I grew up close to the entrance to Lynn Headwaters Regional Park. It is joined to Seymour Demonstration Forest, forming 15,000 acres of parkland on Vancouver's North Shore. With hundreds of miles of winding trails through evergreen forest and varying terrain, they are truly a runner's paradise. I did about 80 percent of my running there and the other 20 percent in Vancouver's legendary Stanley Park, which has about 1,000 acres of forest and trails surrounded by ocean beaches.

Writing *The Thrive Diet* took only as long as I needed to type the words (which was a long time because I'm a slow typist, but that's beside the point). The overall premise of the book had been written in my mind while I was

exercising. Each day after I returned from a run or bike ride, I would write down the central ideas that had popped up in my brain. Within a few months, I had all I needed for the core of the book. From there, I simply (and in some cases not so simply) expanded on each major point and organically evolved the book.

Finding Your Sweet Spot

big-picture ideas are easier to develop during physical activity

I did discover, however, that there's a sweet spot with exercise and the creative process. More exercise is not necessarily better. Your optimal amount depends on several factors. One is fitness level. The fitter you become, the more exercise you can perform before getting fatigued. Physical fatigue is always closely followed by mental fatigue, and once you are mentally fatigued, your ability to generate free-flowing thought and creativity will be greatly hindered or snuffed out altogether. The idea with physical exercise is to stimulate the brain, not cause it significant fatigue. So while longer bouts of exercise are helpful for the creative process itself, the fatigue that follows reduces the ability to apply that creativity. For example: If my morning run ends up being much longer than an hour and a quarter, once finished I'll be too relaxed. Complacent even. That feeling is nice, but the contentment that comes with it is, of course, not conducive to a productive day. It's too satisfying, and as a result the drive to work hard is lessened. And due to the extra physical exertion and resulting mental fatigue, I'm ready for a nap by three in the afternoon—which is fine when you train full-time, but not ideal if you're trying to draw as much as you can out of your productive self. But less is also not necessarily better. The point at which my mind begins to wander varies, but it's usually around the 40-minute mark. So if I exercise for 30 minutes, I achieve neither the desired brain stimulation nor the optimal level of relaxation. I may even feel agitated for the rest of the day, which is not ideal for productivity either.

It will take a bit of trial and error, but you will discover your sweet spot, when exercise complements your productivity by poising your body for the day and allowing your brain to shape its thoughts into ideas and solutions. Someone who has never consistently led an active lifestyle may initially need just a 15-minute walk each morning. A steady buildup of physical activity will lead to improved overall results. On page 80 I provide an Adaptation program to help you begin

an injury-free workout. Suggestions for beginning an injury-free running program start on page 84.

Left Brain, Right Brain

There are two halves to the brain, and each of us tends to favor one side more than the other. The left brain is used for tasks that require a sequential, linear, analytical approach. Following a standard set of rules to solve a math problem is an example of left-brain problem solving. People who are left-brain dominant tend to use logic to solve problems.

Conversely, the right brain is used for holistic, random, big-picture-focused, and intuitive thought. Those who are right-brain dominant have a greater interest in aesthetics, the arts, and music and focus on big-picture ideas, patterns, and creativity. They create from the top down. Seeing the big picture, they build with that in mind.

Defined as the process of making unexpected leaps, creativity is not a linear process. Like any thought, creative thought can be stimulated and channeled during activities that lend themselves to a wandering mind. Swimming, running, and cycling all stimulate the right brain. But if you are not quite ready for these activities, you can start by walking.

Several years ago, while I was on a book tour, I sustained a running injury.

Because I had no races on the horizon and my schedule was packed, I felt okay about taking a little time off from daily exercise to give my body a chance to heal. But by the third day I was having a harder time than normal making decisions and was not thinking as clearly. I didn't have my bike with me, and there were no swimming pools nearby. So the next morning I decided to walk for exercise. Though the mental effect was not as pronounced as with running, I certainly noticed a positive response.

Generating Creativity

> physical activity can help
> us make better use of our
> right brain's attributes

Experts who study the field of creative thought say that we all have the capacity to think in a grand, abstract way. Some people inherently have a greater amount of creativity than others, but most of us could make better use of what creativity we do have. We just have to figure out how to stimulate our creative spark and have it ignite into accessible, readily flowing ideas.

Writing my first book presented a creative challenge for me. From the start, I wondered how other writers dealt with a creative dry spell. Some authors appear to have the ability to churn out high-quality, creative prose day in, day out. Newspaper columnists, for example, write and submit their articles just hours after the event takes place in order to get it laid out, printed, and delivered to front doors across the country the following morning or posted online within minutes. What is that seemingly elusive creative spark that appears to come and go, not following any noticeable pattern? Paradoxically, I found the answer in someone who has discovered the ability to apparently summon creativity at will.

I met Dan Piraro at a social event one summer evening in New York City. Not only has this artist mastered and made significant use of his creativity, but he appears to do it every day. Dan Piraro is the man behind *Bizarro*, a syndicated comic in hundreds of daily newspapers worldwide. Dan has to come up with an original, witty comic every day. He can't afford to have a prolonged mental dry spell; his job and reputation hinge on his ability to overcome creative roadblocks and to constantly produce. So how does he do it? That's exactly what I asked him. His response: "I hop on my bike and ride around Brooklyn. Ideas simply begin to flow. When I arrive home I write down all the thoughts that came to me. From there I weave them into solid ideas and ultimately *Bizarro*. Often I'll

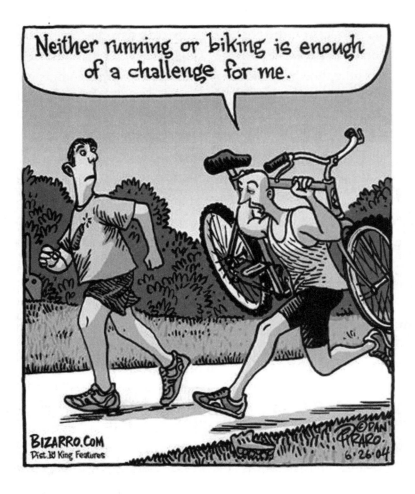

be able to amass two weeks' worth all at once, just from one ride."

Dan's words were reassuring to me. Even the creative elite, who appear to produce with machinelike regularity, go through creative peaks and valleys, just like the rest of us. What separates peak achievers from the rest is their ability to take control of the creative dry spells that will inevitably crop up at some point. Having the ability to stimulate the right brain, thereby drawing what new ideas we can from it, may be more important than possessing lots of pure creativity itself.

Mental Outsourcing

The left brain is responsible for performing linear, sequential calculations based on a set of rules—the kind of thinking computers are good at. If we let technology perform many of these duties for us, if we "outsource" our left-brain responsibility to computers, we free up both halves of our brain for other thought processes.

For example, following a map and making sense of driving directions is the job of the left brain. If we plug the address of our destination into a GPS, we reduce our brain's workload. For those who are left-brain dominant, this creates an opportunity to allow their mind to wander and focus on cultivating their right-brain attributes. And for those who are right-brain dominant, it allows them to do what they do best: come up with big-picture, abstract plans. Instead of focusing on which exit you have to take, you may come up with names for characters in that novel you've always wanted to write. While we can't rely on machines to carry out our right-brain tasks for us, we can, to some extent, delegate to them our left-brain tasks.

I find, however, that the ideas that flow through me when I exercise are just as quick to leave as they are to arrive. I therefore make an effort to remember the sensible ones until I'm done exercising. I used to attempt to mentally store the information and enlist the help of my brain to keep it all straight once I got home. But recruiting the brain to remember information that can be easily written down is a poor use of mental resources. Now I just write the informa-

tion down immediately—and then I can forget it. Finding out that I can get a pad of paper to do a job that normally I'd use my brain to do was refreshing.

It's akin to having the chief scientist at NASA fill his days with cleaning the cafeteria floor while he should be figuring out how to put humans on Mars.

Releasing Endorphins

for greater creative functioning, give your brain a break

Endorphins are brain chemicals released during exercise that reduce pain, improve the ability to fall and remain asleep, and induce a feeling of well-being and happiness.

Athletes can use the pain-reduction effect of the endorphin release to their advantage. Toward the end of a long, hard race, athletes are able to push themselves to the brink; the endorphins that their body releases dull the physical pain to a mild discomfort, enabling them to exert themselves beyond their usual pain tolerance. This is one reason why the day after a race, the competitors are barely able to walk.

Athletes and those who are physically active consistently report a higher level of happiness than their sedentary counterparts. A recent Duke University study on clinical depression conducted on 156 people found that 60 percent of those who exercised 30 minutes three times a week, for 16 weeks, were able to get rid of their depression without using medication. The researchers speculated that this was a result of two different effects of endorphin release. People with clinical depression are thought to have a neurotransmitter imbalance, and endorphins may help to correct this. And people with depression tend to have low energy—but at the same time are unable to consistently get a good night's sleep. The endorphins released during exercise improved their sleep quality.

But it's not just people with clinical depression who benefit. Reports show that endorphins released during exercise can also help those with situational depression. Feeling better (even if it's simply due to a chemical release in the brain) is the first step to being able to identify, acknowledge, and address the situation that is causing them to be depressed.

> endorphin release can help you feel better and therefore perform better

Yoga and meditation are among the best-known and oldest forms of using the body as a means to boost mental health. In general, North Americans who do yoga or meditate regularly are in better health than those who don't. However, this statistic can be somewhat misleading, since North Americans who practice yoga and meditation are usually more health conscious to begin with, they are less likely to eat a Standard American Diet, and their income is higher. Their lifestyle as a whole contributes to their health, not just the fact that they practice yoga or meditate. However, that said, yoga and meditation can do something important for anyone seeking better mental health. And what's interesting is that it's not what we get that is of benefit, it's what we don't get: excess information.

Select Information Diet

Normally thought of as a good thing, information is in fact a problem in modern life. There is simply too much of it, most of it useless. And harmful. Yes, harmful. You may think you can just ignore useless information, but it occupies space in your consciousness and thereby slows the rate at which you can make use of information you actually need. Think of a computer's memory being filled and cluttered up by a constant bombardment of spyware downloads, resulting in a reduced processing speed.

If we retain only important information, the brain will be better able to process that information, make sense of it, solve problems, and allow the subconscious room to work. Yoga and traditional meditation result in restricted information intake and thereby give your brain a well-deserved break. Active meditation in the form of running and cycling provides an opportunity for the brain to mull over information it already has, while restricting entry of new information. No need to go on an information fast—a select information diet will enhance your brain's ability to form thoughts, make connections between ideas, solve problems, and think clearly under stress.

Active Meditation

time during the day that is
not spent consuming information
can be used to bolster mental
health and productivity

When we engage in sports that require quick thinking and extreme focus, we are less likely to be able to slip into the creative realm. While the increased blood flow to the brain can help us reach a meditation-like state, the very nature of these sports makes it difficult *not* to focus on anything. Focus is, of course, direct, specific thought, which is the opposite direction of where we need to go when trying to tap into the subconscious. A parallel can be drawn between the way in which the brain functions during meditation and being physically active while relinquishing focus. Active meditation, as it's appropriately called, has many of the same mental benefits offered by traditional meditation. Most people find active meditation easier to get into due to the increased blood flow in the brain.

physical activity combined
with meditation yields
unique health benefits

Increased blood circulation within the brain can in part be credited for the improved ability to function and delve into creativity. Blood carries oxygen and nutrients to feed the brain. The region of the brain responsible for complex reasoning and concentration, the frontal lobe, has been shown to significantly benefit from more freely and rapidly circulating blood. Increased blood flow to the frontal lobe on a regular basis has also been shown to reduce the risk of two neurodegenerative conditions, Alzheimer's and Parkinson's.

Building Neurotransmitters

While sports that require quick thinking, focus, and coordination do not lend themselves to creative-thought production as readily as repetitive-movement sports, they do in fact help stimulate and even change part of the brain. When the brain learns new movements that require coordination and targeted concentration, it changes physically by making new neurotransmitters. Constant learning therefore helps prevent neurodegenerative disease by keeping the brain active and in a constant state of development and construction. Any new learning is helpful, yet learning new exercise routines is of superior value, since it generates greater blood flow while a new way of thinking is being formed. The combination is complementary and augments brain health. However, once someone has become proficient at the new exercise and can do it seamlessly, without thought, the benefit to the neurotransmitters declines. But if a new exercise is introduced, that brain growth is maintained.

Additionally, on a biochemical level, exercise has been shown to stimulate the production of brain chemicals that encourage the growth of new nerve connections. It is thought this may explain why athletes have lower rates of neurodegenerative diseases such as Alzheimer's and Parkinson's.

Choosing Your Activity

Examples of repeat-pattern aerobic activities, which stimulate the right brain and therefore creativity after proficiency is reached:

Biking
Hiking
In-line skating
Rowing
Running
Speed skating
Swimming
Walking (briskly)

Examples of continually changing movement activities, which increase brain activity until proficiency is reached:

Basketball
Hockey
Racquetball
Squash
Table tennis
Tennis

It makes sense to become proficient at one or two of the repeat-pattern activities from the first list that you find most enjoyable. Using them as your base aerobic exercises will serve you well. Physically, they ensure your cardiovascular system remains in peak condition. Mentally, they bolster your creativity, improve your memory, and enhance your problem-solving ability.

learning while being active maintains and builds brain health throughout life

The continually changing movement activities from the second list require constant thinking, coordination, and planning ahead, which also help build neuroconnections. The goal here, however, is never to become too good at any of them. Once the brain has learned the new skill to a level of comfort, these cerebral benefits diminish. These activities are still of benefit, however, since information changes throughout the activity, and the brain must think, make decisions, and tell the body to do it.

HIGH NET-GAIN NUTRITION

Understanding Body Fuel

Soon after I made the decision to at least attempt to become a professional athlete, I began to investigate the benefits of nutrition. Knowing that I'd have to do a huge amount of training if I was going to be successful, I wanted to ensure I began with the most effective program. I looked at the training programs of some of the top professional Ironman triathletes in the world, with the intention of mimicking their routines. To understand what separates the best from the average, I also looked at training programs of average-performing amateur triathletes. What I found surprised me.

The average athletes' programs differed very little from those followed by the elite. If training discrepancies are minimal, then what causes some athletes to become great while others remain average? As I discovered, training isn't the

AT A GLANCE

- Physical exercise offers a vast array of non-physical benefits.
- Being active can bolster creativity and help develop big-picture ideas through right-brain stimulation.
- Regular exercise can improve subconscious function and problem-solving ability.
- Mental outsourcing can improve mental performance.
- A select-information diet and active meditation can improve brain function.
- Learning new physical movements contributes to the construction of neurotransmitters and therefore may reduce the risk of neurological diseases such as Alzheimer's and Parkinson's.

only factor. In fact, the most significant difference has little to do with training. It has to do with recovery. The difference between average and breakthrough performance is mostly determined by the rate at which the body can regenerate from physical training. On reflection, this made perfect sense. Since training is really nothing more than the breaking down of muscle tissue, athletes who can restore muscle tissue the quickest will have an advantage. They will be able to schedule workouts closer together and thus train more than their competitors. Over the course of a few months, the extra workouts will translate into a significant performance gain. Of course, quick and efficient cellular regeneration is of value to non-athletes as well, because the everyday wear and tear of regular life also breaks down cells.

rate of cellular recovery is the largest contributing factor to peak performance

Once this concept solidified in my mind, cellular regeneration became my focus. I found out that nutrition has the greatest impact on recovery: Food choices can account for up to 80 percent of the total recovery process. Having a newfound appreciation for diet, I began to take mine more seriously. Nutrition itself had never really interested me. But the high-energy lifestyle that proper nutrition can provide was unquestionably something I wanted. If cleaning up my diet was an integral part of becoming a professional athlete, as I speculated it might be, I wanted to know everything I needed to know about it.

I researched nutrition extensively over the years and eventually developed my own nutritional philosophy. It's simple: Improve nutrition to reduce stress, because stress is the root cause of just about all ailments, from minor irritants to major diseases. Initial symptoms of stress are poor-quality sleep, general fatigue, and the desire to eat sugary foods. If you don't address the cause of each of these symptoms, they will progress into body fat gain, inflamed joints, and mental clutter. If these are allowed to continue, they will likely result in one variation or another of cardiovascular disease, type II diabetes, arthritis, or osteoporosis.

I called the resulting nutrition program the Thrive Diet and published a book about it in 2007. The Thrive Diet is extremely effective when adhered to in its entirety, but it does not require an all-or-nothing approach. Incorporating even just a few elements of the Thrive Diet will significantly improve the results of Thrive Fitness.

Did you know you have the ability to grow a younger body? Regular exercise encourages the body to regenerate muscle tissue more rapidly and actually keeps it in a constant state of regeneration. If the cells have been constructed recently, the body is biologically younger. But the body needs high-quality building materials to construct those new cells—in the form of high-quality nutrition.

> regular exercise and
> high-quality food collaborate
> to build a biologically
> younger body

If you live Thrive Fitness, high-quality nutrition will improve the results. Exercise breaks down muscle tissue. With rest and proper nutrition, the muscle grows back stronger than it was before the exercise broke it down. That is the training effect. However, the training effect can be significantly boosted if nutrition is not only complete, but also timed correctly. When you eat is almost as important as what you eat. I explain this in detail on page 145.

What Is High Net-Gain Nutrition?

Since a calorie is a measure of food energy, you understandably might assume that the more calories you consume, the more energy you will have. But if that were the case, people who eat lots of fast food would have boundless energy.

And they don't. The missing element is net gain.

The *net gain* of food is the term I have given to the energy and usable sustenance we are left with once digestion and assimilation of the nutrients have taken place. Foods with a high net gain are whole, plant-based, alkaline-forming foods that are nutrient dense and easy to digest, so that our body can easily assimilate and use the nutrients. (Animal-based whole foods—organic, free-range meat and wild fish—are highly acid-forming and therefore not considered of high net gain.) A diet based on these high net-gain foods—as opposed to simply supplemented with them—will yield impressive health results. A diet based on low net-gain foods, on the other hand, leads to increased physical strain and stress, general fatigue, and cravings for sugar and starch. Not only that, the greater quantity of energy expended through digestion and assimilation will simply leave us with less.

As I mentioned earlier, in relation to energy expenditure during exercise, if you don't spend it, you still have it. If the body is left to decide, it will likely choose to use that energy to improve immune function and quicken restoration of cells damaged by stress—essentially, anti-aging activities.

When we base our diet on high net-gain foods, we gain energy through conservation as opposed to consumption. As you might expect, the first results of such a diet will be more energy immediately following a meal. Unfortunately, most commonly consumed foods in the average North American's diet require almost as much energy to assimilate as they provide. (Note that the nutritional value of food listed on the label pertains to what is in the food, not what net gain the body actually gets from it.) When we eat highly processed foods, fatigue sets in not long after because of all the energy the body must exert in digesting that food. But when we eat high net-gain foods, we can sustain an even energy level throughout the day. This will reduce the desire to snack on unhealthy foods. We won't need to—or want to—consume as many calories when eating a high net-gain diet. It won't take long for our body to respond to the high levels of nutrition and the reduced number of calories. Energy goes up, body fat goes down.

consumption of high net-gain foods conserves energy, resulting in more energy

While we can all benefit significantly from a body that operates more efficiently, athletes have the most to gain. This is because humans cannot function efficiently above a certain core temperature. The extra energy that must be generated and spent to digest and assimilate refined foods as raises the core temperature. The lower the core temperature starting point, the longer the athlete can exercise at a greater intensity before reaching that maximum optimal core temperature. All other factors being equal, a lower operating temperature allows us to perform more work (higher intensity exercise) before experiencing fatigue.

But that's not the only advantage. Let's look at an example. If two runners are equal in every respect except for their core temperature, the one with the lowest temperature has the advantage. Because Runner A is farther from reaching his body's maximum temperature, he can speed up, going ahead of Runner B while expending no additional effort. In addition, because Runner A is farther below his maximum temperature, he perspires less and thus dehydrates less quickly, thereby further enhancing endurance. And because his body does not have to exert as much effort, his heart doesn't need to beat as fast. As we saw earlier, a lower heart rate means that the body has to expend less energy to maintain physical workload. Therefore endurance will be even further improved.

Nutrient-Dense Foods

By consuming more easily assimilated foods, we can conserve energy and reduce stress. Foods in their natural, nutrient-dense state can be digested and assimilated with less energy expenditure. When we eat nutrient-dense, natural foods, we don't need to eat—or digest—as much as when we eat less nutrient-dense foods. In addition, when we feed the body the nutrients it needs, the brain "turns off" the hunger signal.

Raw Foods

Foods that have not been heated above 118 degrees Fahrenheit are termed raw foods. There are several performance advantages to eating a large quantity of raw food in place of its cooked counterpart. Ease of digestion and assimilation, which directly translates into additional energy by means of an increase in net gain, is the most significant. Enzymes that contribute to overall health and aid digestion are not present in cooked food; heating above 118 degrees Fahrenheit destroys them. Therefore, before the body can turn cooked food into usable fuel, it must produce enzymes to aid in the digestion process. A healthy person can create these enzymes, but it costs energy and therefore creates a nominal amount of stress. Enzyme production diminishes with age, leaving us solely reliant on diet to acquire them. In fact, if enzyme-rich foods are not the base of our regular diet, our enzyme production system will have to work overtime and can actually become overtaxed and weakened later in life. Including enzyme-rich foods in our diet on a regular basis will help safeguard our bodies' ability to manufacture enzymes. Interestingly, a person who cannot produce digestive enzymes and does not obtain them through food can acquire the same diseases as someone suffering from malnutrition.

While enzyme quality will sharply drop off at only slightly above 118 degrees Fahrenheit, the next significant quality decline in food will come at a temperature of about 300 degrees Fahrenheit. This is the point at which essential fatty acids convert into trans fats. Additionally, food cooked at a high temperature can cause inflammation. When sugar is heated to a high temperature with fat, it can create end products known as AGEs, which the body perceives as invaders. The immune cells try to break down these end products by secreting large amounts of inflammatory agents. If the cycle continues, it can result in problems commonly associated with old age: less elastic skin, arthritis, weakened memory, joint pain, and even heart disease.

Alkaline-Forming Foods

enzyme-rich foods help ensure the body makes optimal use of the nutrients in the food

The pH is the measure of acidity or alkalinity. Within the body, maintaining a balanced pH is an important part of achieving and sustaining peak health. If our pH drops, our body becomes too acidic, adversely affecting health at the cellular level. People with low pH are prone to many ailments and to fatigue.

The body can become more acidic through diet and, to a lesser extent, stress. Since our bodies are equipped with buffering capabilities, our blood pH will vary to only a small degree, regardless of poor diet and other types of stress. But the other systems that have to be recruited to facilitate this buffering use energy and can become strained. Over time, the result of this buffering will be significant stress on the system, which will cause immune function to falter, effectively opening the door to a host of diseases.

Low body pH can lead to the development of kidney stones, loss of bone mass, and the reduction of growth hormone, which results in loss of lean muscle mass and increase in body fat production. And since a decline in growth hormone production directly results in loss of lean muscle tissue and the acquisition of body fat, the overconsumption of acid-forming foods plays a significant role in North America's largest health crisis. But food is not the only thing we put in our bodies that is acid-forming. Most prescription drugs, artificial sweeteners, and synthetic vitamin and mineral supplements are extremely acid-forming.

Low body pH is also responsible for an increase in the fabrication of cell-damaging free radicals and a loss in cellular energy production. Free radicals alter cell membranes and can adversely affect our DNA.

> an alkaline body has
> significantly higher odds
> of being a healthy body

In addition, viruses and bacteria thrive in an acidic body, which can lead to a wide variety of diseases. Did you know that it is impossible for cancer to develop in an alkaline environment? When acid-forming food is consumed, starting with digestion and continuing until elimination, it produces toxins the body must deal with, because they lead to premature aging through cell degeneration. Highly refined and processed, denatured foods produce toxins and have no usable nutrients, yet they retain their caloric value—the worst combination.

Athletes in peak training are the most affected by acidic body pH. Already physically stressed, many athletes also suffer various types of mental stress such as performance anxiety. Increased metabolism further lowers pH. Since acidity is a stressor, cortisol levels rise, resulting in impaired sleep quality, thus further exacerbating the problem.

Vigorous exercise creates stress in the form of muscle trauma. Physiologically speaking, hard exercise is a stressor, and rest and recovery turn that stress into fitness gains. Athletes require protein and alkalizing foods to help their muscles regenerate. The correct balance of exercise stress and recovery is the recipe for growth.

Cortisol and the Elimination of Biological Debt

Biological debt is the term I use to describe the unfortunate, energy-depleted state that most North Americans live in. Often brought about by eating refined sugar or drinking coffee to gain short-term energy, biological debt is the ensuing energy "crash."

There are two types of energy, one obtained from stimulation, the other from nourishment. Generally speaking, the more a food is processed, the more stimulating it will be to the nervous system. When we consume caffeinated beverages or refined foods, we get energy almost instantly. But it is short-term, unsustainable energy; the stimulation of

the adrenal glands is inevitably followed by fatigue. In our culture, we tend to use additional stimulation to overcome this fatigue, which in turn produces more fatigue, and so on. In contrast, when we eat natural and whole foods, our body is less stimulated and more nourished. Energy derived from good health, so-called cost-free energy, does not take a toll on the adrenal glands, nor does it regularly need to be "stoked" with stimulating substances. People who are truly well have boundless energy without reliance on stimulants such as caffeine or refined sugar.

Stimulation places demand on the adrenal glands and therefore causes production of the stress hormone cortisol. Elevated cortisol is linked to inflammation, which is a concern for the athlete. Higher levels of cortisol also weaken cellular tissue, lower the immune response, increase risk of disease, cause body tissue degeneration, reduce sleep quality, and are a catalyst for the accumulation of body fat.

> stimulation always
> results in fatigue

In *The Thrive Diet* I describe my first exposure to significantly elevated stress levels. I was training too much, and my body could not regenerate quickly enough to support the pace at which I was breaking it down. To make matters worse, I had not yet made the connection between stress production and nutrition, and my diet was average at best. A high amount of physical stress coupled with nutritional stress resulted in an elevated cortisol level, which remained high for an extended period. After about four months, my stress problem had become chronic. I displayed all the telltale signs, but, not understanding the relationship between stress and hormones, I ignored the general fatigue, difficulty sleeping, irritability, mental fog, and cravings for sugar and starchy food. While these symptoms of too much stress were bothersome, they weren't nearly as debilitating to me as an athlete as those that followed. I actually began to gain weight. And it was all fat. I was getting fatter, even though I was training 35 to 40 hours per week. I didn't realize why at the time, but the reason became clear later. Because of my chronically elevated cortisol level, my adrenal glands had become fatigued. So fatigued that they were completely burnt out.

But exercise is not the only cause of adrenal fatigue and exhaustion. Adrenal fatigue, the first step toward adrenal exhaustion, and almost always caused by excess stimulation, is one of the greatest problems facing those of us who live and work in a fast-paced environment. Affecting 90 percent of North America's population, it has reached epidemic proportions. After overconsumption, the greatest reason for obesity in North America is that we are simply inundated with more stress than we can deal with in a sustainable, healthy manner.

Maybe you've seen them, people who come to the gym week after week, month after month, and even year after year but never seem to get leaner. Despite consistent exercise, they can't lose extra body fat or reshape their body. As I discovered firsthand, the underlying problem may be too much stress—from several sources—which culminates in a variety of health problems.

too much stress results in fatigue and body fat accumulation

The solution? Stop exercising. Taking time off from training can be one of the best ways to kick-start results. In some cases, it's the only way to get back on track. The reason these people don't make any gains is that their cortisol is elevated. And because exercise is a form of physical stress, it elevates those levels even further. Rest, eating a high net-gain diet, avoiding foods and drinks that stimulate the adrenal glands, and reducing stress in other areas of life will help bring down cortisol levels, at which time exercise can be reintroduced. When overall stress levels are low, that's when significant exercise gains are made.

Sometimes, however, lightly stimulating foods such as yerba maté, green tea, and matcha can be consumed to yield a significant boost in athletic performance. But afterward, the athlete will have to take appropriate steps to recover from this extra adrenal stimulation. Following the nutritional guidelines in this book will help you stave off adrenal burnout. A particularly beneficial food to help keep the adrenals functioning at their peak is maca (see page 143). I provide pre-workout recipes for boosting workout performance on page 151 and recipes to speed recovery and help the adrenals repair on pages 160 and 164–166.

Principles of the Thrive Diet

To sum up, the Thrive Diet is based on foods that are

- raw or cooked at a low temperature
- naturally alkaline-forming
- high in nutrients that are usable by the body without having to be converted
- nutrient-dense and whole
- rich in vitamins and minerals (rather than supplements)
- non-stimulating

When you transition to a new way of eating, start gradually and build slowly. Remember, even positive change is perceived as stress by the body. By progressively incorporating new elements into your current diet, you will allow your body to physiologically adapt. By avoiding a change-related stress response, you will make a healthy diet desirable and doable.

Depending on your starting point, after about two weeks, your body will adapt and you will see that the results are worth the effort. Over time, your body will actually begin to crave high net-gain foods and lose interest in refined, processed ones. By making high net-gain foods a large part of the diet, you will simply have no room for those other foods. The body will get all the nutrition it needs from the new diet and will turn off its hunger mechanism.

EFFICIENT SLEEP

A Good Rest Is Half the Work

As I mentioned earlier, one of the greatest concerns of the professional athlete is lack of training. This often leads to the fear of not being fit enough, which is then usually countered with more training. Naturally, this results in overtraining. In an effort to help alleviate athletes' fear of rest and help them understand that training is only half the equation for fitness improvement, many coaches began to use this line: A good rest is half the work.

Sleep Builds Strength

Physiologically speaking, training actually reduces the strength of the athlete. At the end of a hard workout, when the most muscle tissue has been broken down, the athlete is weakest. But once muscle tissue is broken down by exercise, the body will grow it back stronger to be able to cope with the demands placed upon it. This is the basic premise of physiological improvement: The body's overcompensation for stress stimulates strength gains. In other words, the high-return exercise you engage in during the day breaks down muscle tissue cells, which the body then regenerates to produce stronger and younger cells, using the energy from the high net-gain foods you consumed.

Your body regenerates muscle cells in the deep phase of sleep, when growth hormone is released. High-quality sleep therefore amplifies and expedites the benefits of an exercise and nutrition program. But if stress levels, and hence levels of the hormone cortisol, are too high, the body will physiologically not be able to get into this deep phase of sleep.

growth hormone release helps build muscle and reduce body fat

Provided that cortisol levels are relatively low, your body will start releasing growth hormone (GH) between 30 and 60 minutes after you fall asleep. Produced in the pituitary gland, GH is known as a powerful anabolic stimulus and thus provides several health-enhancing benefits. As the name suggests, it aids growth. Muscle tissue, tendons, ligaments, and cells in general that have been broken down during the waking hours, and in particular as a result of exercise, are repaired. Growth hormone also renews skin cells, resulting in greater elasticity, which in turn creates softer, more supple skin. And GH stimulates the breakdown of fat cells, which results in body fat loss.

How quickly we recover from exercise is in part dependent on the body's ability to release GH. During times of particularly heavy training, some athletes have a mid-afternoon nap of at least one hour to encourage their body to release an extra hit of growth hormone. And some suggest that GH release can be increased simply by setting the alarm to go off every two hours throughout the night. The rationale: By reaching that 30 to 60 minutes point in the sleep cycle more often, we encourage the body to release GH more often.

Success of course hinges on the athlete's ability to fall back to sleep soon after being woken up by the alarm.

Foods high in starch or sugar will inhibit the release of GH if eaten within 90 minutes of going to bed. In general, it's best not to eat at all when bedtime is near, with one exception: If you are trying to gain muscle mass, you may want to consume half a serving of Vega One mixed with water. Its low starch and sugar content will not inhibit GH release, and the substantial amount of protein, essential fatty acids (EFAs), and fiber will cause the nutrient release into the bloodstream to be slow and prolonged, thus preventing the body from going into a catabolic state (which breaks down body tissue) while sleeping.

high-quality sleep reduces the desire to overeat

Sleep Reduces Appetite

There are two other hormones whose levels depend on sleep quality. Ghrelin, secreted by the stomach, is responsible in part for initiating the sensation of hunger. Leptin, released by the fat cells, signifies satiety to the brain. Levels of ghrelin become substantially elevated when you are tired, and at the same time, the release of leptin is inhibited, with the result that you feel hungry even when your body is, in fact, satiated; you can no longer judge whether you've consumed enough food. Therefore, it is common for people in need of quality sleep to feel hungry. This leads to over-eating and eventually weight gain.

lack of high-quality sleep causes premature aging

Prolonged lack of deep sleep also causes a decrease in the body's ability to use carbohydrate for energy. The first effect is reduced energy levels, since carbohydrate is the body's primary fuel. The second is that, since it is not burned as fuel, carbohydrate is converted to and stored as fat.

Long-Term Effects

People who continue to lack deep sleep face symptoms usually found in those who are considerably older, because lack of deep sleep hastens the aging process. The immediate symptoms are reduced short-term memory, weight gain due to the inability to efficiently metabolize carbohydrate, and even type II diabetes if poor-quality sleep is prolonged.

As we saw in the diagram on page 20, sleep is an integral part of overall health. We need deep, high-quality sleep to allow our body to repair itself while we sleep, and to feel rested, have energy, and avoid sugar and caffeine cravings when we're awake. For a high-quality workout, we need to be well rested and have a sound recovery—both of which are dependent on sleep and nutrition.

How do we make ourselves sleep well? By lowering cortisol levels. That means eliminating as much uncomplementary stress as possible by engaging in high-return activity, eating high net-gain food, and living a low-stress lifestyle.

Quality not Quantity

While some people suggest that most of us should aim to get more sleep, I say the opposite. For the sake of productivity, the less sleep we can get away with, the better. Those extra waking hours give us more time to achieve our goals—provided, of course, we're alert and functioning at a high level, both mentally and physically. In order for that to happen, we need to be well rested. So, although sleep is a central component of health and wellness, it is not the duration that is of utmost importance, it's the quality.

In the modern world, the line between being awake and being asleep has become blurred. Many people spend their days in a state that borders on being asleep. Even after eight hours of sleep, they wake up feeling both physically and mentally tired. And it shows. Their brain wants to get going, so it sends them a chemical message to drink caffeinated beverages and to eat sugary foods. The brain knows that this will help stimulate the body into action. But the effects of caffeine and sugar wear off after a short time, and the result is greater fatigue. Why is this pattern of poor-quality sleep followed by daytime fatigue so common? Stress from lifestyle, but mostly stress from the food we eat. Nutritional stress is caused by the refined foods that are commonplace in the North American diet but also by what could be argued to be a greater problem—the lack of nutrient-dense whole foods.

quality of sleep is more important than duration

There has long been a debate about what's more important for peak health—nutrition or sleep. On one hand, nutrition provides your body with building material to replace aging cells with new, vibrant ones and to reconstruct body tissue. A high net-gain diet also reduces nutritional stress. On the other hand, high-quality sleep is when that repair actually takes place. And high-quality, deep sleep can only occur when cortisol levels are low. Since high net-gain nutrition reduces stress, a healthy diet improves cortisol levels and thus the quality of sleep. Better-rested people do not crave sugary and starchy foods, since they simply do not require their stimulating energy. High-quality sleep thus makes it easier to maintain a healthy diet.

UNCOMPLEMENTARY STRESS REDUCTION

With North Americans reporting steadily escalating incidence of stress-related illness, saying that stress has become an epidemic is putting it mildly. Minor symptoms that occur only days after we surpass our stress threshold can quickly lead to fatigue, difficulty sleeping, and sugar cravings. In the long term, stress can make you ill. While nutritional stress makes up a large proportion of overall stress, there are several lifestyle situations that can create a stress response.

But not all stress is bad. Stress can be divided into three categories: uncomplementary, complementary, and production stress. If we are mindful of these three kinds of stress and their causes, stress is in fact not as difficult to curtail as you might think. You will be able to selectively reduce unbeneficial types of stress while cultivating the kinds of stress that will benefit your life and help

you achieve your goals. (I also present more detail on each stress and its origins in *The Thrive Diet*.)

Three Types of Stress

Uncomplementary stress is any stress that does not provide a benefit. Examples include eating food that lacks nutritional value, breathing polluted air, or worrying about things you have no control over.

Complementary stress is stress that benefits you mentally or physically in some way, such as moderate exercise.

Production stress is stress created in the process of achievement. Examples include working hard on a project that is stressful, yet having something to show for it once it is complete, or engaging in high-level training for sport in excess of what is healthy, yet benefiting by achieving greater fitness.

The body has what I call a stress threshold. Once we go beyond it, we may develop overall fatigue, trouble sleeping, headaches, and sugar and starch cravings. Reducing all types of stress will alleviate these symptoms of general stress in the short term.

You may be stressed from overwork and having trouble sleeping because of your elevated stress hormone levels. Although quitting your job to bring down your cortisol levels is probably not an option, a reduction in workload will lead to a reduction in stress and hence cortisol levels. But how do you reduce stress while maintaining a productive life? Especially if you are a high achiever, the last thing you want is to sacrifice productivity in an effort to lessen stress.

The question is, Can we significantly reduce our stress yet maintain our productivity? I'm pleased to say the answer is yes. Nutritional stress is a form of uncomplementary stress that we can eliminate: If we eat well, we bolster our productivity and vitality.

In fact, when done correctly, calculated stress reduction can significantly boost productivity in the long term. A reduction of uncomplementary stress allows us to engage in more complementary and production stress–promoting activities. For example, if we reduce uncomplementary stress through proper nutrition, we have the opportunity to engage in the complementary stress of exercising regularly without fatigue. This will result in greater fitness and all the benefits that come with it. Lower levels of uncomplementary stress can also give us the vitality we need to take on exciting projects that will likely require hard work and therefore cause considerable production stress. But with

less total stress, we can embrace these projects. To achieve goals we have set for ourselves, there are times when production stress will need to be high. To avoid reaching our stress threshold, we must eliminate stress from other areas.

Willpower Can Run Dry

As I describe in *The Thrive Diet*, willpower can become depleted. It is important to understand the value of this concept when you start a training regimen. Consistently doing things you don't enjoy causes stress. So if you have to force yourself to get through each session, the value of your training is greatly diminished.

In a study on willpower, two groups of children aged seven and eight engaged in very different activities. One group was taken to the beach and allowed to play all day. The kids splashed around in the water, built sand castles, flew kites, and basically just acted like kids. The other group spent the day inside a classroom doing schoolwork. But not just any schoolwork. Each child was forced to study his or her least favorite subject. To make matters worse, the children were each carefully supervised by an adult with the aim of relentlessly keeping them on task.

At the end of the day the groups were each led into separate rooms and asked to sit at a table. Unbeknownst to the children, the researchers were able to watch them through a one-way mirror. One of the researchers then entered each of the rooms in turn, putting a bowl of freshly baked cookies on the table. Both groups of children were told that the cookies were not for them. They were asked to please not touch them and told that the adult would return in a few minutes. With that, the researcher walked out of the room.

The group that had a fun, sunny, and enjoyable day at the beach chatted quietly and barely acknowledged the presence of the cookies. The classroom group, on the other hand, were fixated on the bowl. They squirmed, sat on their hands, and made faces of frustration. They kept creeping closer, a couple of them leaning in to inhale the smell. Then a little poke with a finger, a little piece broken off and eaten. Within 15 minutes, their cookies were gone—eaten by every single one of the children.

> doing what you dislike for a prolonged period of time depletes willpower, making any challenge you take on more difficult

As the researchers suspected would happen, the beach group members were able to exercise their willpower. Because the beach group had spent the day doing exactly as they pleased, the children's resolve was not taxed, and they therefore had a full supply when confronted with a situation that required it. The classroom group had their willpower depleted in the classroom earlier that day by being forced to do things they specifically disliked, and which therefore created a stress response. They simply used up their reserves of willpower and had none left when it was called upon.

We've all been in situations when we have pushed ourselves for an extended period, to the point where we're unhappy and near-exhausted; there comes a point when we need a break. Having the ability to push through no matter what may be helpful in the short term, but in the long term, it makes anything we attempt harder.

Exercise You Enjoy Replenishes Willpower

If you've always perceived exercise as easy and fun, exercise will serve as a willpower restorer after a long day of work. But if you force yourself to do daily exercise that you don't like, it will deplete your willpower, making it increasingly difficult to seek out and take on new challenges. Conversely, if you have to force yourself in other aspects of life, you are less likely to be successful at switching to a new diet or sticking to an exercise program. Many cite their reason for not sticking to an exercise program or eating healthily as simply not wanting to—despite being aware of the vast benefits. Fortunately, the solution is simple.

People who no longer have the willpower to stick to an exercise program are best not to start one. Not right away. They first need to introduce an element into their life that brings them true enjoyment. Maybe you dislike your job. You come home in the evening having burned all of your willpower, and find it very difficult to motivate yourself to exercise. Changing jobs so that you are happier during the workday and have the willpower to exercise in your leisure time may not be an option. The solution? Stop trying to exercise for now and find something you love to do after work. It will fill up your reservoir of willpower. Once you have regained enjoyment in your daily life, you can start exercising. Even though it may not be enjoyable at first, the endorphin release will help enhance your mood and make sticking with it easier.

reduce stress to improve drive and determination

I was once asked by an interviewer for a magazine, "How are you able to constantly push yourself so hard in training and during Ironman competitions?" I had never thought about it. My instant response was, "I don't push myself, I just let myself go." And it was true. I had never viewed what I did as "pushing myself." In my mind, I was doing what I wanted and letting myself go. It was easier for me to train and race than to not. I perceived it as a low-stress, fun activity; therefore, it was easier for me to do than for someone who had to push himself through every workout. And my steadily improving results reflected that.

When you are selecting a recreational activity, pick one you'll enjoy. It's not so much the activity itself as the way you perceive it that is important. For many people, yoga is an excellent form of stress relief. But if you don't like yoga, performing it in an effort to get healthy will have little value and can actually create more stress than it alleviates.

Consider your likes and dislikes, and aim to find a form of exercise that suits your personality. Do you prefer solitary or social sports, vigorous or gentle, competitive or non-competitive, individual or team, indoor or outdoor?

If you want to use exercise to clear your mind after a challenging day at work, a run or walk by yourself may be a good choice; if you want exercise to be your time of the day, away from others, solo activities are the way to go. If, however, you like the camaraderie and social aspect of exercising, choose an activity such as an aerobics class or circuit training. If you need motivation to exercise, arrange to work out with a friend. If you schedule your exercise like any other meeting, you will quickly get into an exercise routine and be encouraged to stick with it.

spending mental energy wisely yields improved productivity

Do you like vigorous activities, such as boxing, or are you more suited to introspective movements, such as yoga? Do you prefer competitive activities to keep you motivated or is competition a turn-off for you? If you flourish with head-to-head competition, try tennis or squash. Do you like team sports? Consider joining a local soccer or ultimate league. Or, if you prefer indoor team sports, try the local volleyball or basketball court. Check with your local recreation center to see what it offers. You will be amazed at the diversity of activities available.

This, of course, isn't limited to sports. You can only fake it for so long before your willpower simply runs dry and you are forced to make a change. Be sensitive to what you like. If you are clear about that, you can offset unpleasant activities with activities that you enjoy in other parts of your life and thus enhance your chance of success. This will build your willpower reserve and allow you to bring to your project a clearer mind and greater ability to work diligently and efficiently.

If you are dreading the thought of having to complete a large project that provides you little interest, recharge your willpower with enjoyable activities. When not working on your project, go out of your way to do things that are especially rewarding to you. Make sure that they are instantly gratifying though; for this compensation mechanism to work, the payoff must be immediate.

being properly nourished reduces stress and therefore builds a reservoir of willpower

In addition to seeking out pleasurable activities, put a hold on doing things you dislike. Since all your resolve needs to be gathered, stored, and released for your project, let other things go and deal with them later. Stop cleaning your house. Seriously. Let go whatever you can. Believe me, you'll be able to retain and unleash more willpower than you had ever thought possible. Your productivity will be unparalleled. (It's a good thing I'm enjoying working on this book or my house would be a mess.)

A mistake I see people make consistently is trying to do too many things at once. Especially when these projects are large, requiring considerable mental resources. You'll improve your odds of success if you focus on one project at a time and pour all your willpower and mental resources into it. It will be completed with greater quality and in a shorter amount of time. Then move on to the next. All the projects you have on the go will still be completed in the same amount of time.

Studies suggest that willpower can be raised by maintaining healthy blood-sugar levels. Willpower is greatest when the body and brain are well nourished. Applying self-control burns blood sugar, which in turn reduces the capacity to further maintain willpower. This is another reason to keep the body well and consistently fueled.

AT A GLANCE

- High-quality nutrition is vital for cellular regeneration and ongoing athletic improvement.
- Regular exercise and high-quality food collaborate in the creation of a biologically younger body.
- Consuming high net-gain foods will result in sustainable, non-stimulating energy.
- The reduction of nutritional stress will significantly reduce overall stress and will boost vitality with no loss in productivity.
- Willpower is finite. When it runs dry, even minor tasks will seem difficult.
- Enjoyable activities restore willpower, resulting in the ability to take on major tasks and overcome significant challenges.

TRAINING, LIVING, AND IMPROVING

Improving continually is as close to
perfection as anyone can hope to get

SHARPENING YOUR FOCUS

3

For the first few years of my athletic career, I was bad at running up hills. For whatever reason, I lacked the proper technique, and my leg muscles had not developed to the point where they could efficiently power up sharp inclines. But I didn't realize it. We all have weaknesses. That itself is not a problem. What is a problem, however, is the tendency for athletes not to recognize their weaknesses. Coaches and others, with the best intentions, will often build the athlete up with praise, only pointing out his or her strengths. Believing that this is helpful and that positive thinking is a component to success can, in fact, allow small weaknesses to remain unaddressed. Pretending everything is fine and glossing over problem areas may be comforting in the short term, but it will not facilitate continual growth. Positive thinking is not all it takes. While I agree that positive thinking has its uses, it can

do more harm than good when it prevents us from seeing and therefore addressing problems.

Once I realized this, I began approaching my workouts differently. Though not quite to the point of telling myself that I was terrible, I did become highly sensitive to my shortcomings. What was holding me back? What was preventing me from running faster and maintaining a quicker pace for an extended period? Were my legs getting fatigued, was my heart beating too fast, or was my breathing at a near-panicked pitch?

being critical of yourself helps you identify weaknesses and fix them

I developed a mental checklist and would go through it each workout to determine my weakest link. If, for example,

I determined that the reason I was unable to raise my pace was because my legs felt heavy and unresponsive, I would make up a workout program aimed at strengthening them. After a couple weeks of implementing the new program, my leg strength had improved by leaps and bounds. Problem solved.

TRAIN YOUR WEAKNESS, RACE YOUR STRENGTH

This is a line I recall hearing on several occasions during my racing days. Basically, it's a way of saying only show your good side and, when no one is looking, fix your problems. Weakness must be exposed before it can be corrected, but the time to be critical of yourself is during training. When you are ready to perform, you can turn off your self-criticism sensor, for it will do you no good on race day and can only serve to weaken you.

JUSTIFIED CONFIDENCE

One of the commonly accepted measures of personal strength is the willingness to identify our weaknesses. If we're not open to exposing our weaknesses to ourselves, we will never be aware of our shortcomings. And we will not be able to establish a plan to fix them. Identifying our weakness will make us stronger—even if we thought we were too strong to have any weaknesses to address.

The result of identifying and eradicating weakness can be referred to as "justified confidence." Being critical of your faults and taking calculated steps to eradicate them is the basis of continual improvement. When you show up to race, you know you are better because you have addressed your problems with real solutions. The confidence that you now exude is genuine and justified, not a false confidence developed through positive thinking. Subconsciously, your brain knows the difference.

For me, this approach has worked tremendously well, facilitating consistent and genuine athletic improvement over the years. The most exciting aspect, however, is that it is not limited to sports and can be applied to any aspect of life.

> identifying and addressing problems is necessary to achieve authentic confidence

PERSISTENCE

Over the past several years, I've had the opportunity to meet many people who, at least by Western standards, have done well for themselves. I grew curious about what, if any, common thread these highly successful people shared. More importantly, could it be learned and applied?

A common attribute did emerge. For some of them, it's an inherent personality trait; they don't even realize they're doing it. Others have had to consciously build and cultivate it as one of their tools. I'm talking about persistence. It sounds so simple, yet it is profoundly effective.

Persistence is one of the most praised traits of people pursuing success—at anything. We've all heard inspirational stories of someone who continually failed at a pursuit, yet persisted undeterred until the goal was achieved. Often the central character in these stories has shortcomings and faults that "humanized" him or her. After facing personal challenges as well as those dished out by the antagonist, our hero persists to overcome the odds.

This notion of persistence is well ingrained in our psyche. We know that if we want something, we have to work hard for it. Interestingly, people who are regarded as highly successful tend to have failed more frequently than the average person. Those who are successful simply try more often; they are the personification of persistence.

There are times, however, when persistence is not the best approach. And it takes intuition to recognize these situations. This is what I believe separates the most successful people of our time from the merely moderately successful. Sometimes, *not* to persist can be the quickest route to success. Sometimes, a change of strategy is in order.

Throughout my high school years, I trained for running and cycling every day. Before school, I would ride my bike at high intensity on a trainer in the basement. After school, I ran in the hilly, wooded trails surrounding our house. Then I'd have a quick shower, eat dinner, do homework (or not), and go to the gym. By the time I arrived home it was about 10 P.M. I would drink a smoothie, go to bed, and get up at 6 A.M. the next day to do it all again. Needless to say, there wasn't much breathing room. Every minute was accounted for to maximize the use of my time; I had traded time for augmented fitness. As a result of this tight program, my running and cycling improved tremendously.

In 1993, I graduated from high school. I was delighted; this meant I could train more. I was going to have time to fit swimming into my program and begin triathlon racing.

I approached swimming with the same vigor I brought to running and cycling: Cram as much in as possible. Since I made significant gains with my running and cycling progress over the previous few years, I figured the more-is-better approach would be the recipe for quick swimming gains as well. I spent hours in the pool each day—for three years. Swimming up to 5.5 kilometers at a time, I was certainly getting fitter. But I wasn't getting much faster.

I was putting in the time, the distance, and the effort but failed to show any noteworthy progress. I added another swim workout, now swimming six days per week and twice on Sundays. I never missed a workout and was the embodiment of persistence. But still no sizable improvement to speak of.

Since I had now dedicated three years to becoming a top-caliber swimmer in the ambition of kicking off my triathlon career with a bang, I grew increasingly frustrated. It was time to try another approach.

I sought the advice of a top-level swimmer. He agreed to make up a swim workout for me, but he insisted on watching me perform it. We met at a local pool. Following a short warm-up in the gym, I hopped in the water and began the workout specifically tailored for me. After I'd swum only one length of the pool, he yelled, "Stop!" I stood up in the pool. "I know what your problem is," he said. "You don't know how to swim."

What? "I've been swimming every day for the past three years," I said in a tone that undoubtedly sounded more than a little annoyed.

He responded by pointing out that, sure, I could swim, but I didn't move fluently through the water, I was fighting every stroke. "Each stroke you make is incorrect. Do you think a golfer would improve if he practiced his swing incorrectly for hours a day, while trying to pack in as many swings as he could and doing them as fast as possible? No, he would ingrain the incorrect movement into his brain. This would make him hit the ball into the bushes every time he teed off. That's what you've done with your swim stroke; you've ingrained the wrong movement."

> persistence solely for the sake of persistence is a poor use of energy

And I realized he was right: I had been doing the same thing over and over to the point of nausea—persevering at all costs in swimming copious distances and finishing every single workout—without evaluating whether it was serving my original goal of swimming proficiently.

That day, I took a step back and re-evaluated the situation logically. Altering my program to focus on the basic mechanics of swimming, and cutting the distance I swam by two-thirds, I slowed down to perform the process of "deprogramming" the cumbersome technique I had inadvertently developed. I replaced regular swim workouts with drill sessions in the water and began to correct my inefficient stroke. After a year of this,

I reintroduced the longer, harder workouts, since I was now moving through the water with a proficient stroke. It, in turn, had become ingrained.

I never did become one of the premier triathlon swimmers, but I did bring about significant gains. And I learned not to persist simply for the sake of persisting. The following year, 1998, I began my professional Ironman triathlon career, with all its 3.8km lake swims.

AT A GLANCE

- Being sensitive to personal faults is necessary in order to identify and eliminate them.
- Positive thinking can do more harm than good and can hinder ongoing progress.
- Building "justified confidence" will significantly help in any pursuit and is only possible once weakness has been determined.
- Persistence is necessary but not the answer to every problem.

PREVENTING AND REVERSING DISEASE

4

SUSTAINABLE HEALTH IS POSSIBLE

As you've read, most diseases that cause a considerable drop in standard of living can be prevented and, in many cases, cured by consistent exercise and sound nutrition. Since the odds of preventing diseases are greater than curing them, living the Thrive Fitness way of life will serve as a strong dose of preventative medicine. In this chapter, I list seven of the most common ailments on which lifestyle can have a profoundly positive effect. Lack of exercise and poor nutrition are directly related to cardiovascular disease and type II diabetes. While genetic factors may play a role for some in elevated cholesterol levels, contracting osteoporosis, and developing arthritis, these diseases are predominantly a result of prolonged inactivity and low-grade diet. Depression and Alzheimer's

are less understood; however, there have been several studies that suggest a diet rich in nutrient-dense whole foods and regular exercise are likely to reduce your chances of developing either of these life-altering conditions.

While the short-term benefits of Thrive Fitness are rewarding, the benefits later in life may prove to be the most valuable.

Arthritis

Arthritis is a disease that affects the joints and usually results in swelling, inflammation, pain, and, in advanced cases, range-of-motion loss. Because symptoms usually don't develop until the disease is advanced (which may take several years), a person may have arthritis but not realize it.

While heredity and impact injuries due to collision will increase the risk of

developing arthritis, these have less in-
fluence than other factors. Fortunately,
the factors that carry the greatest risk
are within our control: lack of physical
activity and excess weight. In fact, the
risk of developing arthritis is cut by up
to 70 percent for people who remain at
a healthy weight and exercise regularly.
From a statistical point of view, living a
lifestyle that will reduce these two risk
factors is the most sensible approach.

Exercise and nutrition help maintain
a healthy weight. And nutrition can help
reduce the symptoms of arthritis as well
as address the cause: People who eat an
alkaline-forming diet will notice a significant reduction in joint swelling from inflammation and therefore improvement
in mobility. A nutrient-packed smoothie
with chlorophyll-rich foods in it, such as
the recipes on page 180, and a large leafy
green salad each day will make a significant difference. The improvements will
be magnified if these alkaline-forming
foods replace foods that cause inflammation, such as dairy, refined wheat
flour, meat, and anything highly processed. When the diet becomes more
alkaline, a reduction in inflammation is
apparent in as little as 48 hours.

Alzheimer's

Alzheimer's, a degenerative disease of
the brain, is the main cause of dementia,
but how it is caused and what drives it to
progress is still largely a mystery. There
is no cure.

As mentioned in the section on
non-physical benefits of exercise, studies
show a link between learning new moves
that take concentration and thought
to perform and a reduction in the risk
of Alzheimer's developing. When combined with exercise, which activates increased blood flow to the brain, learning
has an even greater effect. A sound nutritional approach has also been shown
to likely reduce the risk of contracting
Alzheimer's in the first place. One of
the most helpful preventative measures
through nutrition is thought to be the
regular consumption of foods containing omega-3 and omega-6 essential fatty
acids. Both of these fatty acids are prevalent in hemp, chia, and flax.

Cardiovascular Disease

As I mentioned in Chapter 1, cardiovascular disease is the number-one killer
in North America. When the heart and
the blood vessels become weakened,
the body as a whole suffers. People who
consistently eat fatty animal foods, have
a high level of stress, smoke, and are
sedentary are at higher risk for cardiovascular disease.

The consumption of too much
hydrogenated fat, animal fat, and

cholesterol-rich foods can cause a chronic inflammation of the walls of the arteries (often referred to as hardening of the arteries). Unfortunately, by the time heart problems are detected, this hardening has often progressed to critical levels. If left untreated, a form of cardiovascular disease is almost certain to develop.

The gradual adoption of the Thrive Fitness lifestyle will significantly reduce the risk of developing cardiovascular disease. Foods rich in phytonutrients, such as fruit, vegetables, and chia, are exceptionally good for preventing and combating this disorder. As with diabetes, high-quality nutrition can help slow and possibly stop the progression of disease. So even if you already have cardiovascular disease, changing your diet may help.

Depression

There are two main types of depression: situational and clinical. Situational depression is dependent on external situations that cause sadness. A death of a family member or friend, a divorce, job loss, these can all contribute to situational depression. This form of depression is often easy to diagnose, since there is usually a clear reason for it. Clinical depression, on the other hand, can be very difficult to diagnose and even harder to treat successfully. It is widely accepted by many who study the subject that clinical depression is a chemical imbalance in the brain. What causes that imbalance is largely not understood. Clinical depression can take hold even though life may be perfect. Celebrity magazines are full of stories of people who are rich and famous, who have "made it," yet struggle with bouts of depression.

As I mentioned in the section about the non-physical benefits of exercise, exercise has been shown to help those with depression feel better because it causes a release of endorphins. Once the person begins to feel better, he or she can more easily address the root cause of the problem. Regular exercise has been reported to have an exceptionally high success rate for lessening the severity of the brain chemical imbalance by releasing endorphins.

Elevated Cholesterol

Usually when we think of cholesterol, we think of the bad kind, which significantly raises the risk of cardiovascular disease.

However, there are two types of cholesterol, one of which can be classified as "bad" and the other as "good." The bad cholesterol, also known as low-density lipoprotein and more commonly simply as LDL, can be linked to numerous health conditions. When too much of this type of cholesterol is consumed as part of the diet, it circulates throughout the blood. Over time, it will begin to oxidize and build up under the lining of blood vessels. It will eventually reduce the flow rate of blood, therefore putting greater strain on the heart. If untreated, this can lead to coronary artery disease. It is interesting to note that only animal products contain this type of cholesterol; it does not exist in plant foods. This being the case, the elimination of LDL-containing animal products is the best way to safeguard yourself against all diseases that stem from restricted blood flow through the arteries and blood vessels. They include all types of heart, cardiovascular, and artery disease.

High-density lipoprotein, or HDL, on the other hand, is known as the "good" cholesterol. Raising its level will reduce LDL cholesterol since it acts as a forager of bad cholesterol, collecting it and returning it to the liver for elimination. HDL is also said to have a protective effect on the heart and blood vessels; it serves as an antioxidant as well as an anti-inflammatory and anti-clotting agent.

Consistent exercise will significantly reduce the risk of developing a dangerously high level of LDL. That, combined with eating a plant-based diet, will prevent cholesterol from ever being a con-cern. The reduction of LDL cholesterol is also possible, and is quite easy, with increased physical activity and improved diet. It has been said that aerobic activity will have the greatest impact on the prevention and the reversal of elevated LDL cholesterol. Running, swimming, cycling, or even just brisk walking will be of significant value. A well-orchestrated resistance training program such as Thrive Fitness will also improve muscular strength and thereby remove strain from the heart, which in turn will allow it to deal with restricting blood vessels more efficiently. This will buy time while aerobic exercise is introduced and LDL cholesterol–containing foods are taken out of the diet. Additionally, as a further benefit, all types of exercise have been shown to increase HDL cholesterol.

Osteoporosis

Osteoporosis is a bone disease caused by a reduction in bone mineral density that leads to an increase in fractures. Complications from these fractures can be debilitating or fatal. Its origin can be genetic, or age- or lifestyle-related. Recently, osteoporosis rates in North America have risen sharply. There are two main contributing factors. The first is the unprecedented influx of refined foods in the typical North American's diet, which are not only low in assimilable forms of bone-building calcium but also extremely acid-forming. I explain this in detail on page 132. The second is the widespread reduction in physical activity. Bones remain strong and can be remodeled through exercise—just like muscles. However, when not used on a regular basis, their density tends to decline, leading to low bone density and often osteoporosis. And, to a lesser degree, the fact that life expectancy is rising due to advanced medical procedures also increases the overall number of people with osteoporosis. Of course the longer a person is alive, the greater the odds that he or she will develop a disease of some sort.

The movement of muscles helps strengthen bones, because when a muscle contracts, it pulls against bone. The weight training exercises in this book are an excellent way to increase bone density and significantly reduce your chance of developing osteoporosis. As with any disease, the best approach is prevention. Impact sports such as running build greater bone density in the legs and hips; the bones adapt to all that pounding by increasing their density. If you do not have a running background and already have low bone density, I suggest you start with walking. If you are not more than 20 pounds overweight and can walk briskly for 30 minutes with

no shin or hip pain, you may be able to slowly introduce a running program, using the Adaptation program followed by the running mileage buildup chart on page 85.

Type II Diabetes

Type II diabetes is a metabolic disorder caused by a diminished response to the hormone insulin, which regulates blood glucose levels. The resulting high blood sugar can lead to blurred vision, lethargy, and changes in energy metabolism, and eventually to cardiovascular disease, kidney failure, blindness, nerve damage, and poor wound healing.

Also known as adult-onset diabetes, type II diabetes is a disease on the rise. In fact, the Centers for Disease Control have characterized it as an epidemic, based on the rate at which it has risen and the sheer number of people it now affects. According to the American Diabetes Association, in 2012, 29.1 million Americans had diabetes—i.e., 9.3 percent of the population—and 1.7 million new cases were reported that year alone. Additionally, Health Canada has cited type II diabetes as one of the fastest-growing diseases in Canada, with 100,000 new cases reported yearly, resulting in over 2 million Canadians with the disease in 2014. Prediabetes is even more prevalent, affecting 86 million

Americans in 2014, 90 percent of who were unaware that they had it.

Type II diabetes is rampant in developed nations, and, as with many other diseases, poor diet and low levels of physical activity are a major catalyst. Formerly, only middle-aged and older people were at risk. Now, however, adolescents are developing the disorder at an alarming rate. Lack of exercise and an abundance of nutrient-lacking, insulin-spiking foods are mostly to blame. In general, people who are obese have a significantly higher risk of developing type II diabetes later in life.

What that means is that we have the ability to prevent the disorder—if we break our reliance on highly processed food and foodlike substances and engage in regular exercise.

Living the Thrive Fitness lifestyle will prevent type II diabetes from developing in the first place, but it will also partly reverse the disease if it has already taken hold. Studies show that in many cases, a well-planned exercise program combined with a balanced, plant-based diet will reverse the effects of type II diabetes. Both aerobic exercise and resistance training have been shown to be effective in treating and preventing this disease. When combined, they form a synergistic effect that is of even greater value.

ACHIEVING AND MAINTAINING
THRIVE FITNESS

You'll reap what you sow

PERFORMANCE- BUILDING EXERCISE

5

GETTING STARTED

This is the heart of the book—the applied step-by-step programs to guide you from where you are to where you want to be. Leading off, I've outlined what I feel are the commonly overlooked fundamentals for a successful training program (breathing, warming up, stretching, and hydration). As basic as they may seem, I've learned a few tricks over the years to squeeze every bit of effectiveness from them. For those of you new to exercise and weight training, I've included a detailed Adaptation program. For a fitness program to morph into a way of life, small steps are necessary in the beginning. The Adaptation program will serve as a launching pad for the main Thrive Fitness program.

Perhaps common pre-existing weakness such as lower back pain, rounded shoulders, or knee and shin vulnera- bilities prevented you from immersing yourself in a life of activity. I've included a specific program to correct each of them. This program can also be used preventatively to reduce the risk of weakness developing initially or reoccurring. For running, I've incorporated a specific buildup strategy designed to help you increase mileage and fitness while significantly reducing the risk of injury.

EXERCISE FUNDAMENTALS

Breathing

Believe it or not, many people forget to breathe when they first adopt an exercise program. Best results are achieved when breathing is steady, deep, and in accordance with the pace of movement that the exercise requires. For all the weight training exercises, breathe in when performing the relaxing segment of the exercise and breathe out when lifting the weight.

Warming Up

Warming up serves several purposes. It gently raises the heart rate, which will prepare the body for the more intense exercise to follow without shocking it. It also causes the blood to begin circulating more rapidly so that muscles loosen up and become supple, thereby reducing risk of injury. And once muscles limber up, they work more efficiently, which will allow you to lift more weight and improve faster.

Five minutes of brisk walking, stair-climbing, doing jumping jacks, or even just running on the spot will do. While a warm-up is vital, there are no advantages to a long one. In fact, getting your body accustomed to physical activity in a shorter amount of time can prove beneficial.

I once attended a lecture given by the assistant track coach of legendary British middle distance runner Sebastian Coe. Nearly unbeatable in the late 1970s and early 1980s, he won four Olympic medals and set 11 world records in the 800m and 1500m track events. Reminiscing about Sebastian's training, the coach shared stories of the athlete's glory days. As you might expect, grit, determination, and furious competitiveness were central themes to his anecdotes. But Sebastian and his coach knew that success is not built merely on hard work and brute force; it also requires a systematic, calculated, goal-oriented approach.

> only a short warm-up is needed to benefit the quality of your workout

Many of the middle distance runners of the time were obsessed with the sheer quantity of training, but Sebastian knew better. The others would pack in as much mileage as they could, running for 45 to 60 minutes just as a warm-up before they began their intense track session. Sebastian would be done with his warm-up in 12 minutes. It simply did not take him any longer to be physically warmed up and ready to start the track workout. More running would only have burned more energy and therefore added to his fatigue, which would have reduced the intensity with which he'd be able to perform the key track workout. Sebastian began the workout fresher and therefore got more out of it. This allowed him to improve at a quicker rate. Ever resourceful, while others were trying to see how much longer they could warm up for, Sebastian and his coach were trying to figure out how to whittle the warm-up down further and still have it serve its primary purpose. Eventually, they condensed it into eight minutes. By training his body to become accustomed to warming up faster, he expended much less energy before the actual race than his competitors did. Brilliant.

Stretching

Following a warm-up, a small amount of light stretching can help the muscles limber up and ready themselves for the training session.

BENT-OVER STRETCH

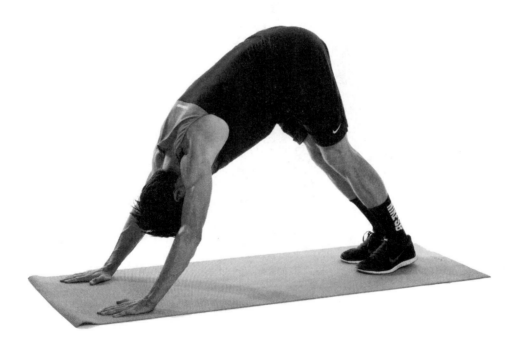

Stand with feet together and bend over, placing your hands flat on the floor, far in front of you, forming a triangle with the floor with your heels still touching the floor. Be sure to maintain a slight knee bend to prevent possible hyperextension and injury. Maintain this position for 30 seconds, breathing deeply the whole time.

Stretches: calves, hamstrings, lower back, upper back

QUADRICEPS STRETCH

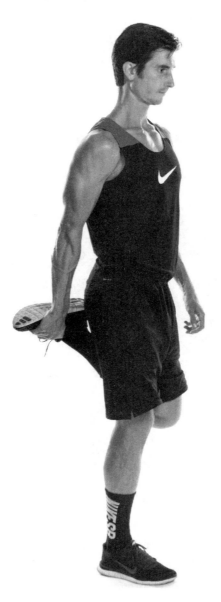

Stand with feet shoulder width apart, bend the left leg at the knee, and reach back with your right arm to grab the upper part of your foot with your right hand. Hold for 30 seconds. Repeat with the right leg/left hand.

Stretches: quadriceps

SHOULDER, CHEST, AND HIP FLEXOR STRETCH

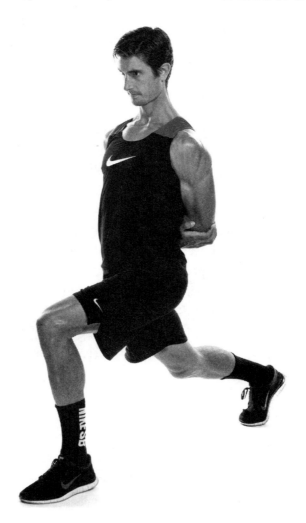

Stand and take a giant step forward with the left leg, so that the lower leg is perpendicular to the floor. Fold your arms behind you, clasping your upper arm just above the elbow with the opposite hand. Exhale fully and tighten the grip on your arms. Inhale slowly and deeply, feeling the stretch through your chest and shoulders. Also feel the stretch through the top of the left leg, at the hip flexor. Hold for 30 seconds. Repeat with the right leg forward.

Stretches: shoulders, chest, hip flexors

Hydration

Hydration plays a vital role in the ability to tap your athletic performance. When muscles are appropriately hydrated, they move fluidly. Not as much energy needs to be spent on muscle contractions, thereby conserving it. Additionally, when the blood is properly hydrated, it will be thinner, enabling its efficient distribution throughout the body. This will result in a lower heart rate and will be directly translated into improved performance. Hydrated cells swell, causing an anabolic response by the release of a growth hormone, therefore speeding cellular renewal. In addition, hydrated cells remain alkaline. If, on the other hand, cells become dehydrated, a catabolic response will ensue. With the release of cortisol due to the augmented stress placed on the heart, the result will be advanced cell degeneration.

Maintaining blood volume through proper hydration allows for efficient delivery of oxygen to muscles by red blood cells, decreased resting heart rate that results in energy savings, stronger muscle contractions by means of anabolic response, effective delivery of nutrients and hormones throughout the body, and removal of waste products such as carbon dioxide and lactate. Each one of these factors will cause workout quality to improve.

Since your body can effectively absorb only about a cup of fluid at once, sipping water or an electrolyte drink throughout the day helps maintain hydration better than gulping large amounts of water only a couple of times a day.

Breathing causes small amounts of moisture to be expelled on each exhale, so it's common to wake up feeling slightly dehydrated and therefore thirsty. Many North Americans begin their day by drinking coffee. Since coffee is a diuretic, feeding it to an already dehydrated body is a biologically straining start to the day. If you just sip water within 10 minutes of waking up, you will replace the fluid that you exhaled over the course of the night. This post-sleep rehydration is especially important when performing a morning workout. Sipping on a sport drink (recipe on page 152) or plain coconut water or coconut water with a bit of lemon juice will rehydrate your body faster than water alone.

THE ADAPTATION PHASE

If you have lacked regular physical activity for the last few years, I recommend you get a medical check-up before beginning Thrive Fitness (or any form of exercise). Remember, change can cause stress, even if it's good change, so build up gradually.

If you have not been physically active so far, suddenly incorporating exercise into your life can result in more cardiovascular strain than is good for you. If your heart is not used to pumping a larger volume of blood, and doing it more rapidly, throughout the body, your arteries may have lost their elasticity, thereby restricting blood flow and placing strain on your heart.

If artery-clogging foods have been a regular part of your diet, the strain on your heart during exercise will be significantly intensified. Following the dietary guidelines in this book and in *The Thrive Diet* will stop further hardening of the arteries and, in many cases, help them regain their elasticity.

As part of the Adaptation program, you may include a form of aerobic exercise such as walking. Begin by walking 20 minutes every second day as a sensible way to ease into it. If walking is bothersome to your joints, try walking on a soft surface such as a grass field. If that doesn't help relieve the strain sufficiently, consider cycling or riding a stationary bike at the gym. The main objective is to raise the heart rate moderately. Once you have built comfort (usually in about three weeks), you can increase the pace—but at this stage in your exercise regime, your walking or cycling should never feel difficult. Once you feel proficient and your level of fitness improves, increase your pace until your heart rate rises to the level that it was when you first began your walking program. As you would expect, your pace increase will parallel your fitness gains.

Whether you've just started being physically active or have been exercising for decades, if you've never weight trained regularly, an adaptation phase is the best way to introduce the routine and ensure that the body can adapt without injury. Not just your muscles, but your tendons, ligaments, and connective tissue in general will be recruited into use during weight training. They will all need to be prepared for the increased workload. Unfortunately, our tendons and ligaments don't adapt to exercise as quickly as our muscles do. Sometimes the muscles gain strength faster than the tendons and ligaments and can therefore lift more weight than what the tendons and ligaments can support. This can lead to tears in the tendons and ligaments, which may take several months to heal.

Following is a gentle approach, designed to allow for adaptation. The number of repetitions for each exercise is higher than that prescribed for the main Thrive Fitness program. When selecting weight, you should feel as though you're capable of performing at least five more repetitions than you will actually complete. The first 10 or so repetitions of each set should feel exceptionally easy. The goal of the adaptation phase is not to push the muscles to the brink but to gently stimulate them.

Even with light weights, it is normal to experience stiffness the following day if you have not lifted weights before. If significant stiffness spills over into the next day that you are scheduled to perform the program again, hold off until it has dissipated.

Adaptation Program

In your adaptation phase, perform the following program three days per week on non-consecutive days. Details on the stretches are on page 75, and the exercises start on page 89.

Warm-up	Duration (in minutes)
Aerobic activity such as brisk walking, jumping jacks, or cycling on a stationary bike	5

Rest between warm-up and stretching: none

Stretch	Hold for (in seconds)
Bent-over stretch	30
Quadriceps stretch	30 (each leg)
Shoulder, chest, and hip flexor stretch	30 (each side)

Main Exercise circuit	Reps
Lat pull in on ball	15
Step back lunges	15 (each leg)
Push-ups with leg to opposite knee	15 (each side)

Core Exercise circuit	Reps
Plank leg lift	10 (each side)
Jackknife on ball	15
Double crunch	15

FIXING AND PREVENTING COMMON PROBLEMS

Lower Back Pain

As any evolutionary biologist will tell you, lower back problems are among the greatest burdens of upright locomotion. Almost everyone I know has, or has had, lower back pain. It is the number-one complaint treated by physiotherapists. The activities of daily life can cause imbalances among the muscle groups that support the lower back—our lower back muscles and our abdominal muscles. These muscle imbalances precipitate lower back pain.

I used to have bouts of lower back pain, but since I started regularly doing the exercises below, they have become very infrequent. It's all about strengthening the core region—the lower back and abdominals—because those muscles act as a protective girdle that stabilizes your lower back. Daily activities will become less efficient physiologically if the core muscles are weak.

A strong core is important for everyday life, but it is vital for peak running efficiency. Each time the foot strikes the ground, energy is transferred up the leg and into the core. If soft, the core will absorb the energy, and therefore not allow it to be transferred back to the ground, which is what moves the body forward.

Since we can't change our way of locomotion, we have to find another solution to lower back strain. Performing these simple muscle-balancing exercises three times per week on non-consecutive days will dramatically strengthen the core, thereby improving efficiency and reducing the risk of pain and injury.

Lower Back Exercises

Complete one set of each exercise in sequence. Complete three sets total. This circuit will take about 10 minutes total.

Exercise	Reps	Rest between sets (in seconds)
Bridge to hamstring curl	20	20
Superman	20 (each leg)	20
Jackknife on ball	15	20
Side double crunch	20 (each side)	20
Double crunch	25	0

Rounded Shoulders

As with lower back problems, rounded shoulders are often caused by a muscle imbalance. Most of us use the muscles of the chest and upper shoulders significantly more than those of the upper back. The shoulders are pulled forward by those stronger muscles. At the same time, lack of use causes muscles in the upper back to become weaker and to atrophy. As the chest continues to get stronger, the muscles tighten and pull the shoulders forward. Leaning over a computer for hours a day is a major contributing cause.

For athletes, rounded shoulders can result in reduced lung capacity. We simply can't breathe as deeply with rolled-in, hunched shoulders. You can test this for yourself by rolling your shoulders in and taking as deep a breath as possible. Breathe out. Now roll your shoulders back and again breathe in deeply. The difference in lung capacity is about 15 percent. Measurable performance gains are made in aerobic sports with a lung capacity improvement of only a couple percent, so imagine what 15 percent can do. Good upper body posture is critical to success in endurance sports.

We need to use a two-pronged approach to fix rounded shoulders. First, improve the flexibility of the chest muscles. This will release some of the tension and allow the back muscles to draw back the shoulders with less resistance. Second, tighten the upper back muscles to pull back the shoulders and have the strength to anchor them in place.

Knee Pain

Knee irritation is a common problem for those new to running. While genetics play a large part in determining whether knee problems will develop and cause pain, there are a few things you can do to minimize the negative effects of all that pounding.

Some people's knees turn in slightly when the foot is pointing directly forward. Somewhat less common are people whose knees rotate marginally outward. Both of these traits increase the risk of running-provoked knee pain. However, with a systematic, holistic approach, the knee area can be strengthened, thereby significantly reducing the risk of knee problems. In addition to proper warm-up, stretching, and the following knee-specific exercises, you may find it helpful to be properly fitted with shoes designed especially for those who are prone to knee pain. Most running-specific stores will have staff that can evaluate your running style and therefore assess which shoes will be appropriate.

My left knee is angled in slightly, and my right one even more so. When I first began running, I was told it was unlikely that I'd be able to run on a regular basis without developing knee problems because of my off-kilter knee alignment. In fact, more than one physiotherapist told me I should find another sport because I didn't have "favorable biomechanics" to be a runner.

I decided to take a preemptive strike and see to it that my knees were safeguarded against injuries due to my poor alignment. I discovered that knee health depends in large part on the shins and the lower back. Following is an exercise program that helped me build and maintain knee strength and mobility, which, in addition to preventing injuries, has brought about greater efficacy and therefore improved performance. With these exercises, I was able to avoid developing even a slight knee irritation.

Increased quadriceps strength has been shown to reduce the risk of knee injuries. In addition to these exercises, you may want to consider working cycling into your regular routine for its quadriceps-strengthening attributes.

Knee Exercises

Hold each stretch for 30 seconds, while breathing fully and deeply. As soon as the first is complete, go on to the next one, also holding it for 30 seconds. Repeat this circuit three times and then move on to the exercises that follow. If you are currently experiencing knee problems, perform this stretching circuit followed by the strengthening program, alternating between four and three times weekly on non-consecutive days. If you don't have knee problems, perform the circuit twice weekly on non-consecutive days as a preventative measure.

Stretch	Hold for (in seconds)
Quadriceps stretch	30 (each leg)
Shoulder, chest, and hip flexor stretch	30 (each side)

Exercise	Reps	Rest between sets (in seconds)
Bridge to hamstring curl	15	20
Step back lunges	15 (each leg)	0
Superman	20 (each leg)	20
Double crunch	20	20

Shin Splints

When I first started running, I got in-jured within two weeks. Like so many novice runners, I fell victim to too much enthusiasm. Shin splints, an injury or inflammation to the muscles in the front of your lower leg or foot, is the most common injury among new runners. If ignored, shin splints can become ex-tremely painful and eventually develop into a stress fracture. That's what hap-pened to me. I developed a stress frac-ture in my left tibia that prevented me from running at all for about a month, and I got a taste early in my career of how unpleasant it is to be injured.

After I'd healed from my stress frac-ture, I found two simple exercises that helped safeguard my shins against fur-ther problems. When I began doing these exercises regularly, in conjunction with the mileage buildup technique (see below), I was able to increase mileage without ever having shin pain again.

Shin Exercise

Do this exercise on non-consecutive days, three days a week, after your run. It takes about 10 minutes to complete.

Stay Injury-Free with Safe Running Mileage Buildup

After my injury, I learned that we need to build up running mileage gradually so that our tendons, ligaments, mus-cles, and bones are able to adapt to the new workload. I had been running more than I was physiologically capable of.

The safest approach is to increase running mileage or time by no more than 10 percent per week and to follow a three-week build cycle with one week of recovery, in which you run half the aver-age of the previous three weeks. The fifth week is the same as week two, and so on. I find that running time is actually easier to calculate than distance. Simply time each run and add up the total number of minutes you spent running in a given week.

For example, if you went for a 30-minute run on Monday, a 60-minute run on Wednesday, a 45-minute run on Friday, and an 80-minute run on Sun-day, your total for the week would be 215 minutes. That means that the fol-lowing week, you should not exceed 236 minutes of running (215 x 1.1 = 236, rounded down). The third week, you

Exercise	Hold for (in seconds)	Sets
Have a towel rolled out in front of you on the floor; with bare feet, roll it up using your toes	20 (each foot)	3

Week #	Mon.	Tue.	Wed.	Thu.	Fri.	Sat.	Sun.	Total maximum weekly minutes
1	30	rest	60	rest	45	rest	80	215
2	30	rest	65	rest	50	rest	91	236
3	30	rest	70	rest	60	rest	100	260
4	rest	rest	40	rest	20	rest	58	118
5	30	rest	65	rest	50	rest	91	236

run for 260 minutes total. The fourth week is a recovery week, so you run 118 minutes (215 + 236 + 260 = 711 ÷ 3 = 237 x 0.5 = 118). Above is a breakdown of the first five weeks of buildup in our example. It's not necessary to stick to the exact minute on each run, but this chart will serve as a general guide.

EFFICIENCY

As an endurance athlete, I've obsessed over efficiency. A seemingly insignificant gain in efficacy can mean the difference between having a professional athletic career and having to get a day job.

You may have seen it unfold on TV—a marathoner or triathlete collapsing just meters from the finish line. Their body has burned all its reserves and cannot go any further. Because so many muscle contractions are performed in an endurance event that lasts several hours, even a tiny amount of energy conserved with each contraction can end up making the difference between victory and collapse.

In the early 1980s, some endurance athletes began supplementing their regular endurance training with weight training, hoping to improve endurance. The results were mixed. Many of those athletes gained some strength, but they also gained weight. Therefore their strength-to-weight ratio showed only very modest improvement—certainly not enough to justify the energy expended on the extra workout. But some of those athletes saw their strength-to-weight ratio drop. Why? They were doing bodybuilding-style workouts, designed to grow muscle size with little or no improvement in functional strength.

A few decades ago endurance athletes were encouraged to avoid "gym training" for fear they would develop heavy, bulky muscles. The reasoning was that extra mass without function will inhibit endurance performance. This makes sense. But that was in an era when gym training was closely associated with the bodybuilding culture. As I explained earlier, bodybuilding does not necessarily lead to increased strength. Bodybuilders lift weights for muscle symmetry and definition, but primarily to build bulk.

When endurance athletes realized that various weight training principles and techniques could be reworked to make bulk-less strength gains, gym workouts once more became popular. But some athletes were not convinced, even though it was now clear that a finely tailored weight training program can build strength without an increase in size or weight. Why would an endurance athlete need strength? And would the results of the extra gym workouts be worth the extra energy expenditure? Would the return on investment be justifiable?

Let's answer that with an example. If two runners are completely equal in every respect except for muscular strength, the stronger one will be faster over any distance. The lower percentage of maximum strength needed for each stride will translate into improved efficacy and therefore greater endurance. If, for example, the one runner can squat 10 percent more weight than the other, his muscles will not have to work as hard to move the body forward, which can translate to significant endurance gains. When muscles don't need to work as hard, they also don't require as much oxygen or circulating blood and therefore will not put as much demand on the heart, which in turn will lower the rate at which it beats. Therefore, this greater strength, commonly referred to as functional strength, does equal greater endurance.

Properly structured gym workouts have now been embraced by most high-level endurance athletes. While the focus for endurance runners and cyclists is the legs, they also work on their upper body. Gains in upper-body strength can translate to a significant performance advantage by improving muscle efficacy. Each time muscles contract, they rely on the blood to provide oxygen and nutrients and remove waste products in the form of carbon dioxide and lactate, so that they can continue moving fluently with ease. While the legs do most of the work, the arms move too. It makes sense to increase the strength of the upper body as well so that it doesn't become too much of an oxygen draw on the system as a whole and thereby increase the heart rate.

The stronger our muscles, the more efficiently they work: Strength equals efficacy. But strength also equals slower consumption of carbohydrate (our muscles' prime source of fuel). For endurance athletes, both elements are crucial. As explained earlier, greater muscular strength directly translates into greater efficiency. Additionally, as the ability to burn carbohydrate more efficiently improves, the longer it will last, thereby further improving endurance.

THRIVEFHIIT AT A GLANCE

Max strength / build / afterburn	
5-minute warm-up (jogging, walking stairs, jumping jacks, etc.)	
Push-Ups with Stands: Favoring One Arm at a Time	Max one arm out at 15 reps, and then the other. Then do as many push-ups as you can in 30 seconds using both arms evenly.
Pistol Squats	Perform 20 reps. Repeat with the other leg. Once complete, do 30 air squats (see page 102).
Lat Pull in on Ball	Perform 15 to 25 reps.
45-Degree Angle Shoulder Press	Perform 20 reps.
Bridge to Hamstring Curl	Aim for 30 reps.
Triceps Press with Stands	Perform as many reps as you can, until you burn out your triceps.
Step Back Lunges	Perform 20 reps on each side (alternating), 40 total.
Plank Leg Lift	Perform 15 reps with each leg (alternating), 30 total.
Superman	Perform 20 slow and controlled reps with each arm/leg (alternating), 40 total.
Jackknife on Ball	Perform 30 slow and controlled reps.
Side Double Crunch	Perform 25 slow and controlled reps on each side.
Strength conversion / power / efficiency	
Warm-up: 30 air squats (see page 102)	
Alternating Ball Push-Up	Perform 30 reps.
Alternating Jump Ground Punch	Perform 20 reps on each side (alternating), 40 total.

continues

ThriveFhiit at a Glance *continued*

Push-Ups with Leg to Opposite Knee	Perform 20 reps with each leg (alternating), 40 total.
Deep Jump Squats with Elbows Thrust Up	Perform 30 reps.
Crab Crawl Push-Ups	Perform 40 push-ups.
Skater Hops	Perform 20 reps in each direction (alternating), trying to string as many together without rest.
V Ups with Weighted Ball	Perform 30 reps.
Surfer Spins with Full Jump	Perform 15 reps in each direction (alternating), 30 total.
Chair Squat Jump	Perform 30 reps.
Mountain Climbers	Perform 30 reps with each leg (alternating), 60 total.
VO$_2$ / lung power / functional strength	
5-minute warm-up (jogging, walking stairs, jumping jacks, etc.)	
Fast Push-Up Knee to Elbow	Perform 15 reps on each side (alternating), 30 total.
Bicycling with Ball	Perform 30 reps on each side (alternating), 60 total.
Alternating Plyometric Lunge	Perform 20 reps per leg (alternating), 40 total.
Roll to Cross with Arms Out	Perform 20 reps on each side (alternating), 40 total.
Deep Squat with Weighted Ball Throw	Perform 25 reps.
In and Out with Arms Parallel on the Ball	Perform 20 reps.
Jump Squat While Lifting Weighted Ball Straight Out and Up	Perform 20 reps.
Double Crunch	Perform 30 reps.
Squat Sidekicks	Perform 20 reps with each leg (alternating), 40 total.
Swooping Cobra Push-Ups	Perform 20 reps.
Plank	Hold plank position for 90 seconds.

THRIVEFHIIT: THE WORKOUT PROGRAMS

I created each of these workouts to individually focus on a specific aspect of fitness. When combined, rounded and complete fitness will be the result.

Max Strength / Build / Afterburn

The purpose of this workout is to build strength, which can later be converted into efficiency, and therefore functionality. This routine will also build lean muscle, which will cause your body to burn fat for hours after the workout is complete; this is known as afterburn.

The goal of this workout is to perform all the exercises in a slow, controlled manner. Your heart rate will stay relatively low, but the muscles being worked will develop true strength that will be converted into functional use with the *strength conversion / power / efficiency* phase.

For some of these exercises, you'll need push-up stands, an exercise ball, or a weighted ball.

5-minute warm-up (jogging, walking stairs, jumping jacks, etc.)
Rotate through the circuit three times. It should last about 45 minutes total, with a maximum 30 seconds of rest between each exercise.

PUSH-UPS WITH STANDS: FAVORING ONE ARM AT A TIME

Equipment: push-up stands

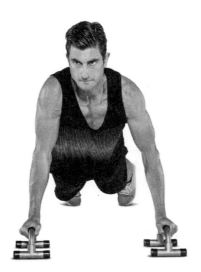
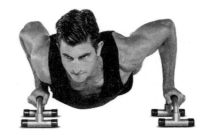

Get in the push-up position, with your arms straight but not locked. Begin with most of your weight on one arm, using the other just for stability. Slowly lower yourself down, taking about 3 seconds to get to the bottom. Pause for 1 second, and then slowly push yourself back up, taking about 3 seconds to reach the top. Continue until you reach 15 reps. As each rep becomes harder, use the balancing arm to assist. The goal is to max one arm out at 15 reps. Once you've finished the first arm, switch so the focus is on the other arm and complete another 15 reps. Then do as many push-ups as you can in 30 seconds using both arms evenly.

Make It Easier: Perform the push-ups on your knees.

PISTOL SQUATS

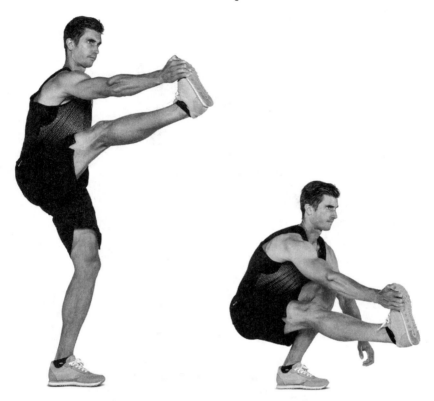

Standing on one leg, extend the other straight out in front of you. Grab your extended foot with the same-side hand, if you can. If your flexibility doesn't allow you to grab your foot, hold your calf. Using the wall for balance and assistance, if needed, slowly lower yourself down until you are hovering just above your grounded foot. Pause for 1 second. Slowly lift yourself straight up, back to starting position. Perform 20 reps. As your leg fatigues, use the wall for greater assistance. Repeat with the other leg. Once complete, do 30 air squats (see page 102).

Make It Easier: Instead of straightening the extended, non-working leg, bend it at a 45-degree angle and only lower yourself to a 90-degree angle, then stand up.

LAT PULL IN ON BALL

Equipment: exercise ball

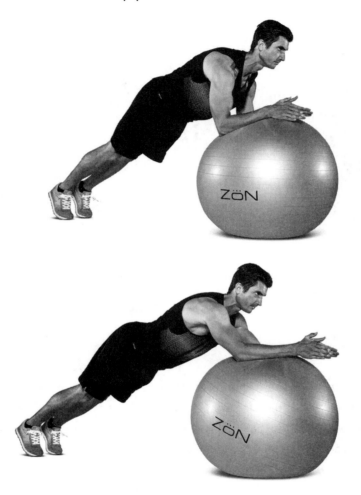

With body straight and core tight, bend forearms 45 degrees and place on a large ball. Your heels should be raised. Keeping the core engaged and the back flat, slowly extend arms until they are straight. Slowly pull them back. Repeat 15 to 25 times. You will feel your lats working.

Make It Easier: Don't extend the arms as far, or perform on your knees.

Make It Harder: Try favoring one arm at a time, and then switch.

45-DEGREE ANGLE SHOULDER PRESS

Equipment: push-up stands

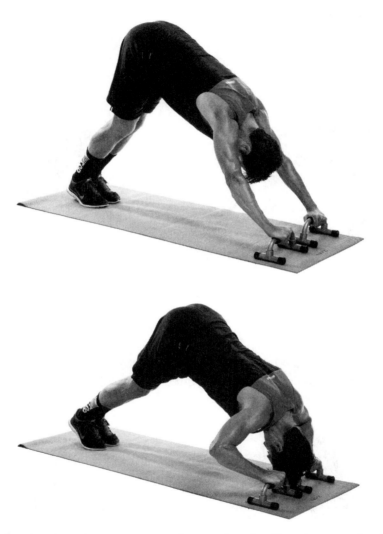

With your hands on push-up stands, walk your feet back so that your body is bent at a 90-degree angle and your weight is on your toes. Your heels should be raised. Slowly lower yourself down with your arms, then push yourself back up. Complete 15 reps.

continues

45-Degree Angle Shoulder Press *(continued)*

Make It Easier: Extend your right or left leg out, raising it off the floor. This will shift your body weight back, reducing the amount of weight that your arms will need to push.

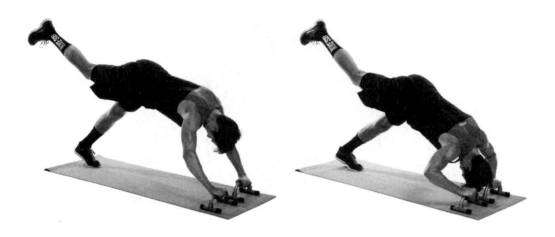

Make It Harder: Bring your right or left leg forward, toward your elbow. This will increase the amount of weight that your arms will need to push.

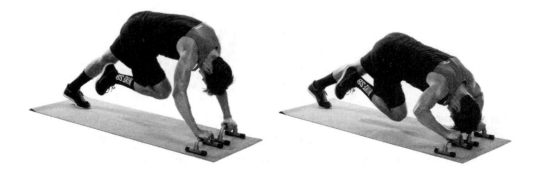

BRIDGE TO HAMSTRING CURL

Equipment: exercise ball

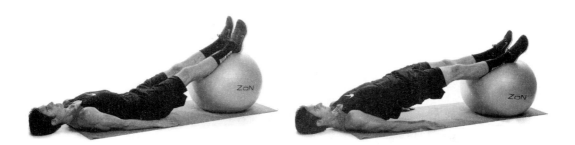

Lie on your back on the floor, bend 45 degrees at the hips, and place your feet on an exercise ball with your legs extended. Place your hands under your head. Slowly straighten your body, so that your hips come off the floor and only your shoulders, hands, and head are touching the floor. Bring the ball toward you by contracting the muscles in the back of your legs. Then push your pelvis up, aligning your legs with your upper body. Keep the movement slow and controlled. Slowly lower yourself back down and repeat. Aim for 30 reps.

> *Make It Easier:* Use your arms for balance by straightening them out and resting them on the floor, parallel to your body.

> *Make It Harder:* With knees bent, put your feet on a bench instead of a ball. This will take away the stability and utilize your core muscles more.

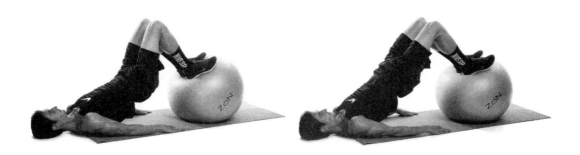

TRICEPS PRESS WITH STANDS

Equipment: push-up stands

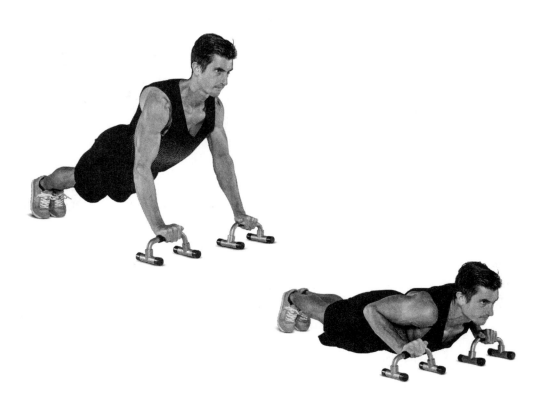

Grip push-up stands with palms facing forward. In a push-up position, with body straight and core tight, slowly lower body down to the floor. Push yourself back up. Perform as many reps as you can, until you burn out your triceps.

Make It Easier: Walk yourself forward, or perform on your knees.

Make It Harder: Walk yourself back.

STEP BACK LUNGES

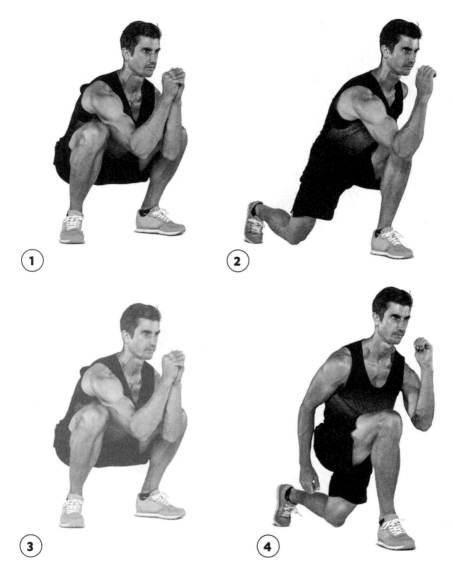

In a deep squat position, with arms bent at about 90 degrees, step your right leg back and, in a running-like motion, bring your right arm up and swing your left arm back, while staying low in squat position. Return to starting position and repeat on the other side. Continue alternating sides until you've performed 20 reps on each (40 total).

PLANK LEG LIFT

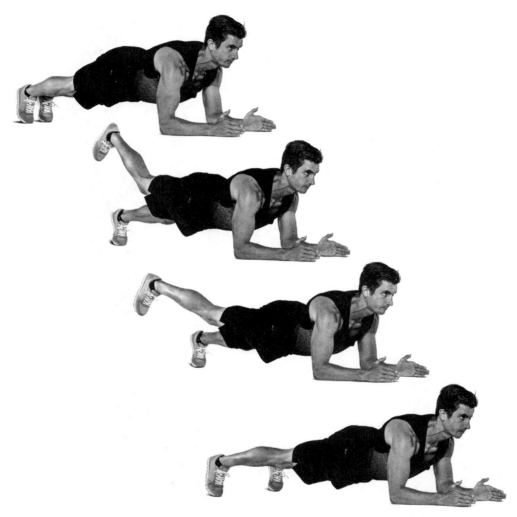

Get in a plank position, with your forearms on the floor and parallel to each other. Keeping your core tight, slowly lift your right leg straight up, bending at the hip. Swing it out to the right, then lower it down and tap the floor with your toe. Raise your leg back up, swing it back in, and return to starting position. Repeat with the other leg, alternating between the two until you've completed 15 reps with each leg (30 total).

Make It Easier: Perform the same motion on your knees.

SUPERMAN

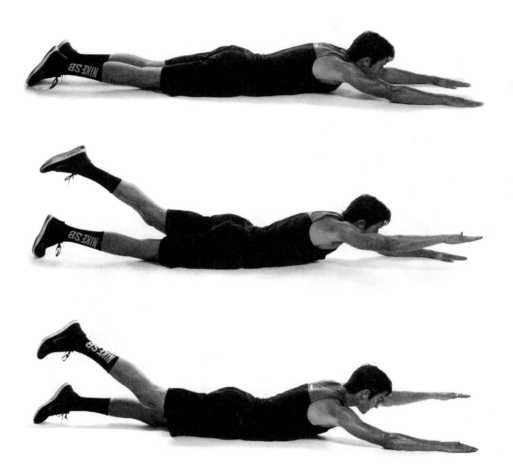

Lie facedown on the floor with legs and arms fully extended. In a slow and controlled movement, simultaneously lift your right arm and left leg. Pause for 2 seconds. Slowly lower back down. Repeat with your left arm and right leg. Alternate until you have performed 20 reps with each arm/leg (40 total).

Tip: *To avoid straining the neck muscles, make sure you do not lift your head too high. Focus your gaze just a few inches in front of you.*

JACKKNIFE ON BALL

Equipment: exercise ball

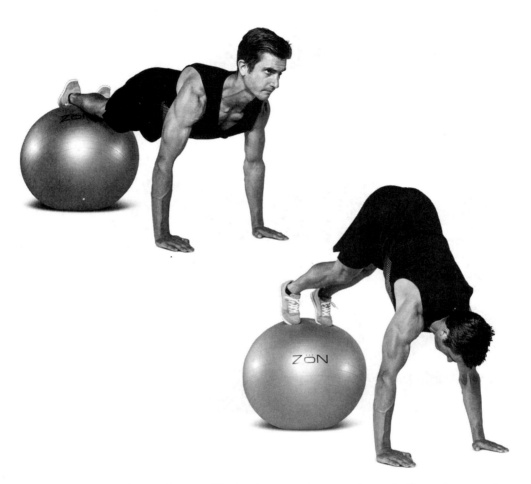

With the front of your feet and lower legs resting on a large ball, get into push-up position. While keeping the core tight, bend at the waist, driving your hips up, and use your abdominals to pull the ball forward. Maintaining tight abdominals, slowly lower back down. Perform 30 slow and controlled reps. It's okay to rest between reps; the main thing is to get them all done.

Make It Easier: Instead of bending at the hips, simply draw the ball forward, keeping your shins parallel to the floor.

SIDE DOUBLE CRUNCH

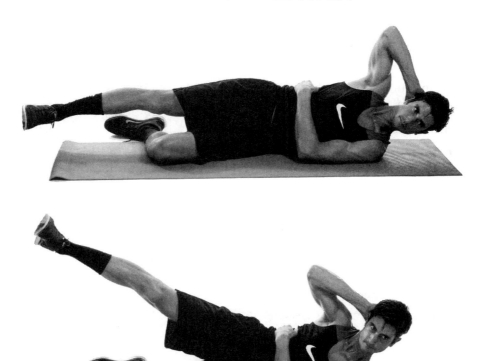

Lie on the floor on your left side, with your left knee bent 90 degrees, your left fore-arm across your chest, your right leg fully extended, and your right hand behind your head. With a slow and controlled movement, simultaneously raise your right leg and draw your right elbow up and over, toward your raised leg. Lower back down. Continue until you have performed 25 reps. Once your set is complete, switch sides and repeat.

Tip: *Make sure not to pull your head with your hand; let the muscles in your sides do the work. Point the toes of your extended leg slightly toward the floor for proper alignment.*

Make It Easier: Bend your raised knee 90 degrees rather than keeping it extended.

Strength Conversion / Power / Efficiency

I designed this routine to convert the strength you've built in the *max strength / build / afterburn* workout into power, which will equate to great efficiency and directly translate into fluidity of movement—and therefore reduced cardiovascular strain during daily activity. This lowers overall stress and all the symptoms related to it, greatly reduces the risk of cardiovascular and degenerative disease, and improves overall health and performance. It is also designed to get your heart rate up and keep it there for the entire workout. Go from one exercise to the next, with as little rest in between as possible.

Rotate through the circuit two times. It should last about 30 minutes total, with no rest between exercises.

Warm-up: 30 air squats
Slowly crouch down into a deep squat and stand up. Repeat.

ALTERNATING BALL PUSH-UP

Equipment: weighted ball

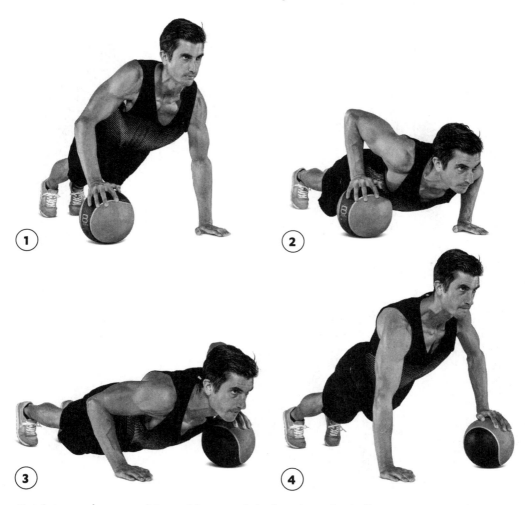

Get into push-up position with your right hand on the ball. Lower yourself down. Push up as fast as you can off of the ball. Roll the ball to your left hand and repeat. Perform this set 30 times. If you're unable to do this 30 times, come to your knees when it becomes too difficult.

Make It Easier: Perform the full set on your knees.

Make It Harder: Push up as fast as you can so that you get air over the ball.

ALTERNATING JUMP GROUND PUNCH

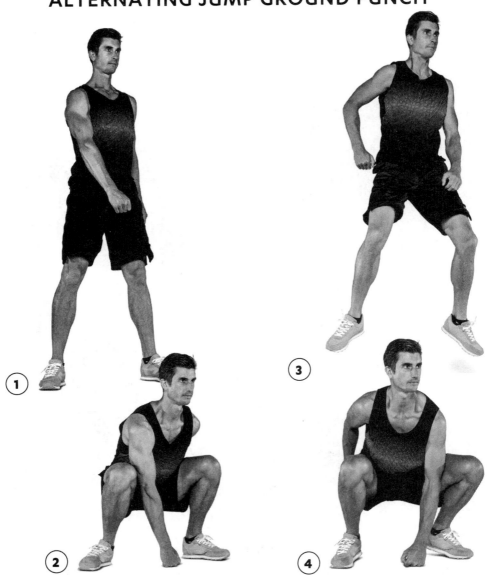

Standing with your feet shoulder width apart and your right hand clenched in a fist, lower into a deep squat, keeping your back straight and making sure your knees don't go over your toes. Put your right fist on the floor. Explode up and come back down with your left fist hitting the floor. Continue alternating fists until you have performed 20 reps on each side (40 total).

PUSH-UPS WITH LEG TO OPPOSITE KNEE

Equipment: push-up stands

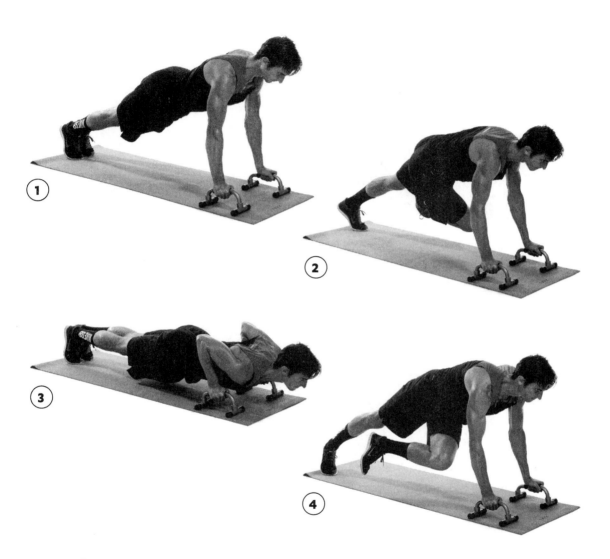

In the push-up position, while keeping your core tight, slowly bring your right leg across your chest, return it to starting position, lower down, and push up. Repeat with the opposite leg. Continue alternating legs until you have performed 20 reps with each leg (40 total).

DEEP JUMP SQUATS WITH ELBOWS THRUST UP

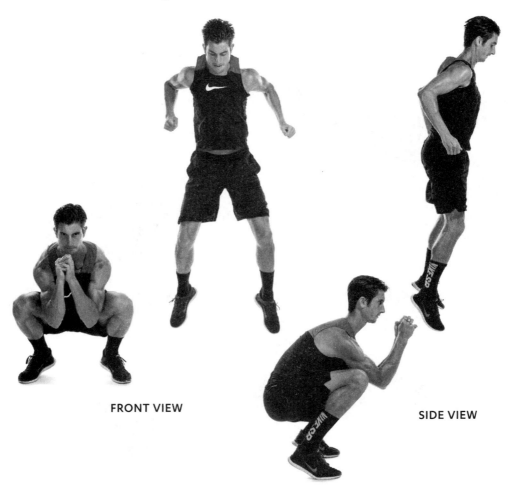

FRONT VIEW

SIDE VIEW

Squat as low as you can. Jump straight up, driving your elbows straight up behind you as an assist. Driving up with your elbows will strengthen the muscles that draw your shoulders back, allowing you to more easily fill your lungs with air. Additionally, driving up the elbows will take some strain off the legs, allowing them to contract more quickly. Since converting strength into power and therefore efficiency is the goal of this workout as opposed to strength building, faster leg contractions are better than slower ones with more weight. Perform 30 reps total. It's okay to rest between jumps, but string as many together as you can before resting. If 30 is too many, do them as quick air squats when jumping becomes too difficult.

CRAB CRAWL PUSH-UPS

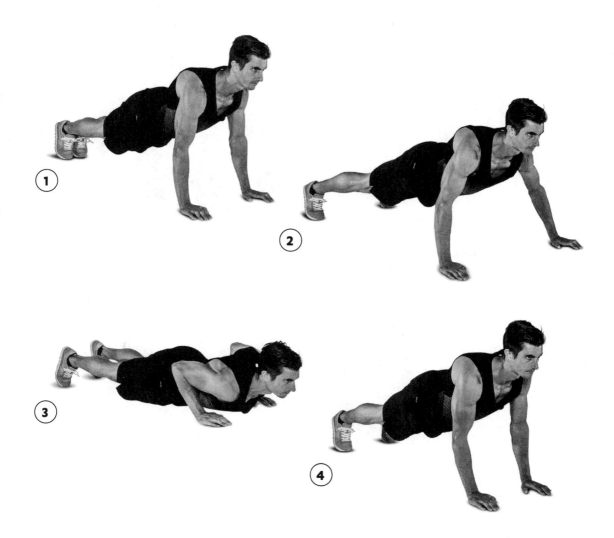

From the push-up position, lower yourself down to the floor, then quickly push up. Move your right arm and right leg out and shift your weight over. Then lower yourself, push up, and step to the left. Return to starting position, then move your left arm and left leg out and shift your weight over. Perform 40 push-ups total.

Make It Easier: Perform the push-ups on your knees.

SKATER HOPS

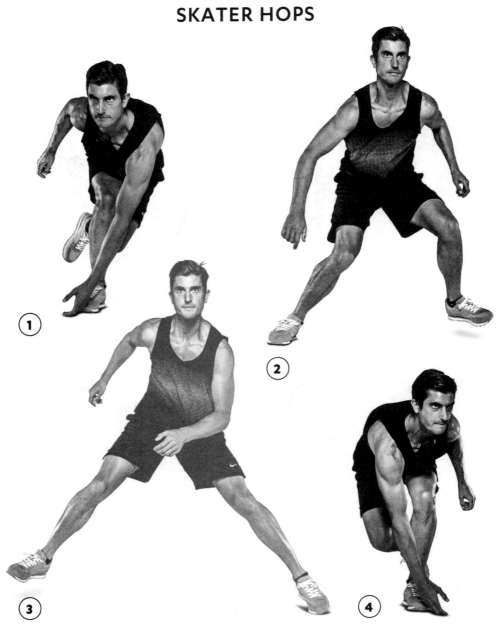

Crouching down with the left leg raised behind the right for balance, push off and leap sideways, landing on the left leg and letting the right swing behind you for balance. Repeat without stopping. Perform 20 reps in each direction, trying to string as many together as possible without rest (40 total).

V UPS WITH WEIGHTED BALL

Equipment: weighted ball

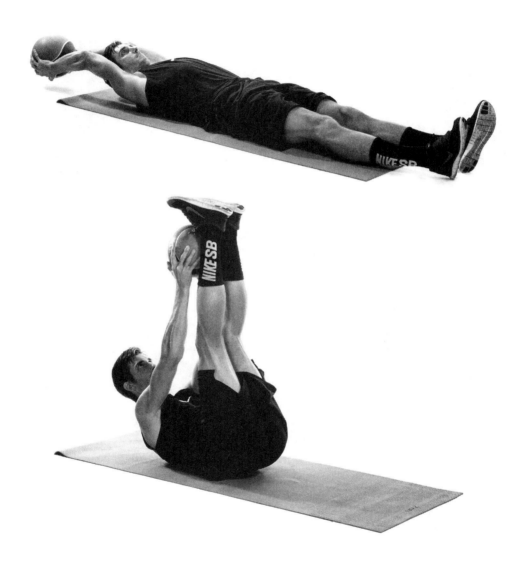

Holding on to a weighted ball, lie on your back with your arms stretched out behind you. Simultaneously, bending at the hips, and bringing your arms up, crunching the abdominals, bring the ball to your feet. Pause for 2 seconds. Return to starting position. Perform 30 reps total.

SURFER SPINS WITH FULL JUMP

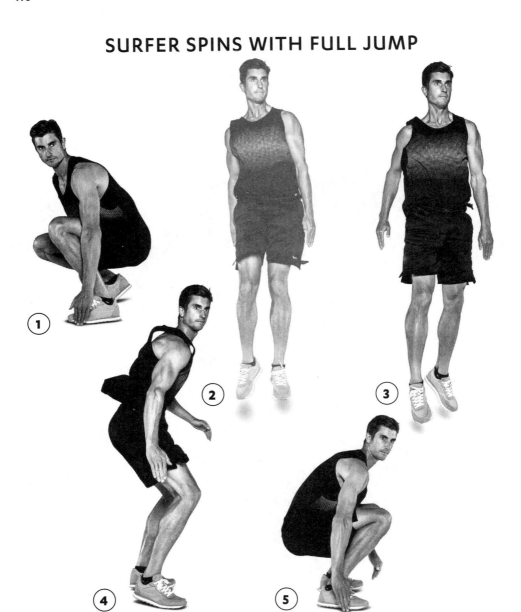

Crouching down with head turned sideways, front hand on the front foot and the other behind you, jump as high as you can, spinning your body 180 degrees while maintaining a forward gaze. Touch the front foot with the front hand while landing. Repeat, spinning in the other direction. Perform 15 reps in each direction (30 total).

Make It Easier: Don't jump as high or squat as low.

CHAIR SQUAT JUMP

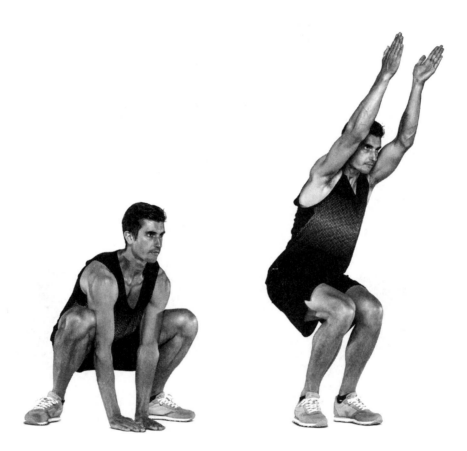

In a deep squat position with palms flat on the floor, hop up, but only so that legs extend to a 90-degree bend (as if sitting in a chair), simultaneously bringing legs together. Perform 30 reps.

MOUNTAIN CLIMBERS

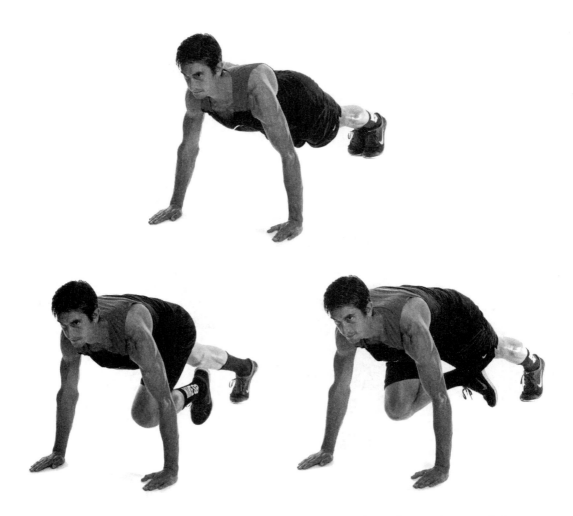

In a push-up position, keeping the core tight, bring one knee forward, toward the chest, then extend it back out. Repeat with the other knee. Continue alternating knees until you have performed 30 reps on each side (60 total).

Works hip flexors, shoulders, core.

Make It Easier: Don't pull the knee in as far.

Make It Harder: Go faster!

VO$_2$ / Lung Power / Functional Strength

The purpose of this component is to boost VO$_2$ max and to teach your body to function efficiently while in oxygen debt. As you'll see, I've structured it in such a way that an intense exercise is followed by a lower-intensity one. The reason for this is to allow the heart rate to drop, thereby enabling it to reach a higher rate during the intense exercise bouts. There needs to be a clear distinction between high intensity and low intensity to get the greatest benefit from this set of exercises. VO$_2$ max training also boosts the ability to efficiently utilize oxygen during any activity and dramatically reduces the risk of developing cardiovascular disease.

5-minute warm-up (jogging, walking stairs, jumping jacks, etc.)

Rotate through the circuit two times. It should last about 30 minutes total, with a maximum 30 seconds of rest between each exercise.

FAST PUSH-UP KNEE TO ELBOW

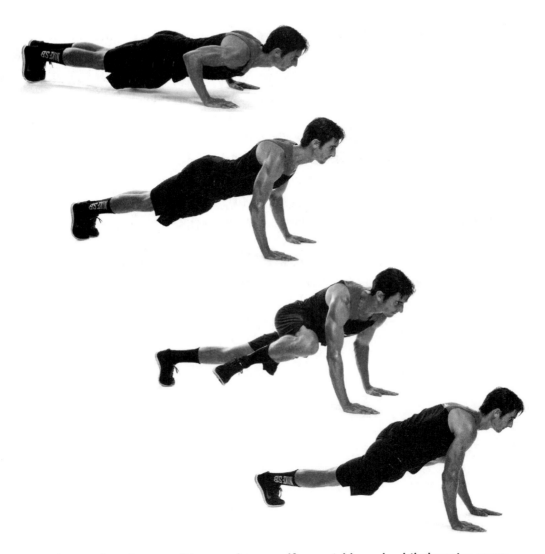

From a lowered push-up position, push yourself up quickly and, while keeping your core engaged, bring your right knee up toward your right triceps. Move leg back to starting position, drop back down, quickly push up, and repeat with the other knee. Continue alternating knees until you've performed 15 reps on each side (30 total).

Make It Easier: Perform on your knees, but maintain the speed.

BICYCLING WITH BALL

Equipment: weighted ball

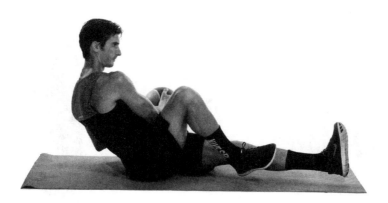

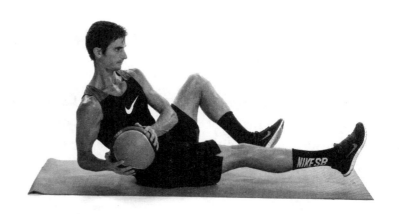

Holding a weighted ball to one side, while keeping the core tight, extend the leg on that side straight out, lifted off floor, while keeping the other leg bent. Twist, shifting ball to the other side while drawing in your extended leg and extending your bent leg. Continue alternating sides until you've performed 30 reps on each (60 total).

Works hip flexors, core, obliques, biceps.

ALTERNATING PLYOMETRIC LUNGE

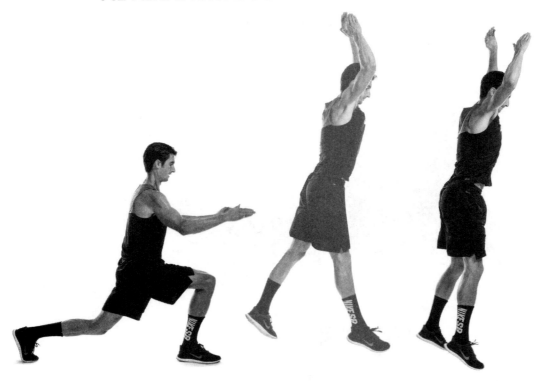

With both arms extended in front of you, with a slight bend at the elbows, one leg bent at 90 degrees and the other extended behind you, explode up, throwing your arms up and switching legs in the air. Continue jumping until you've performed 20 reps per leg (40 total).

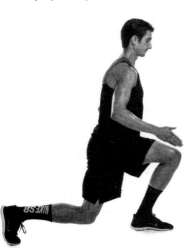

Works quads, glutes, hip flexors, hamstrings, delts.

Make It Easier: Don't drop as low, and slow down the movement.

Make It Harder: Perform faster, and drop deep into each lunge.

ROLL TO CROSS WITH ARMS OUT

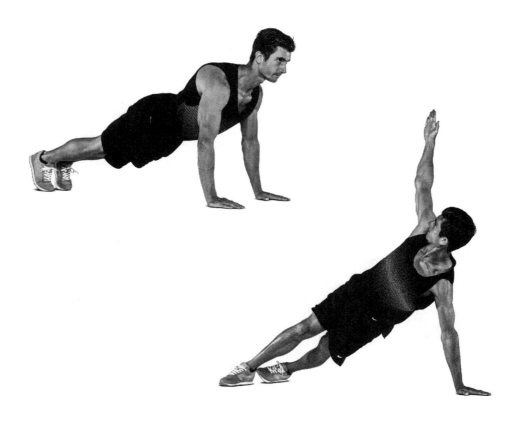

In the push-up position, with your core tight and arms straight, roll out and extend into a cross. Try not to sink down into your hip but keep your core tight. Hold for 3 seconds, then slowly roll back down. Repeat, rolling the other way. Continue alternating sides until you've performed 20 on each (40 total).

DEEP SQUAT WITH WEIGHTED BALL THROW

Equipment: weighted ball

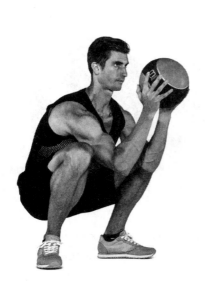

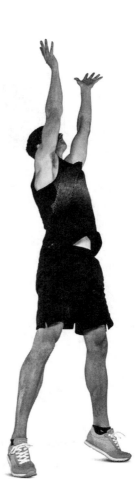

In a deep squat, holding a weighted ball, stand up quickly and rise to your toes, simultaneously pushing the ball straight up into the air as high as you can. Catch the ball while sinking back down to starting position. Repeat 25 times.

Make It Easier: Hold on to the ball throughout the full motion.

IN AND OUT WITH ARMS PARALLEL ON THE BALL

Equipment: exercise ball

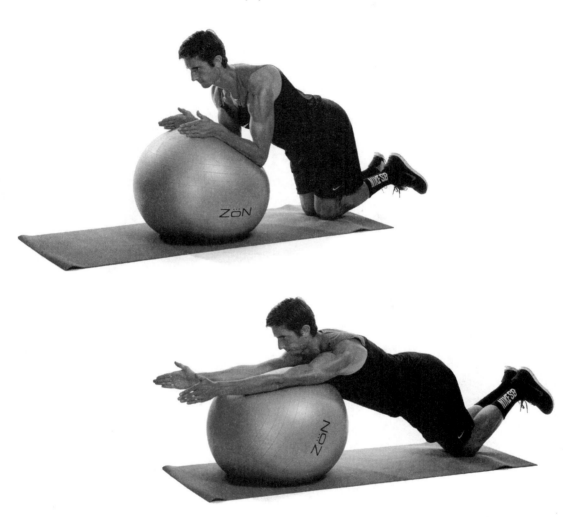

With knees on the floor, place arms parallel, with a 90-degree bend at the elbows, on a large ball. Keeping the core engaged, slowly extend your arms. Pause for 2 seconds. Draw the arms back in. Repeat 20 times.

Make It Easier: Do not extend your arms as far out in front of you.

JUMP SQUAT WHILE LIFTING WEIGHTED BALL STRAIGHT OUT AND UP

Equipment: weighted ball

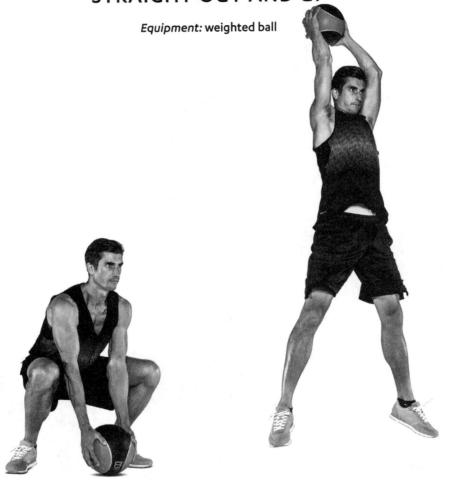

Begin in a crouched position, with arms extended in front of you and holding a weighted ball. Keeping your core engaged, explode up with your legs and thrust your hips forward, simultaneously bringing the ball over your head while keeping your arms straight (or slightly bent). Land and return to starting position. Repeat 20 times.

Make It Easier: Keep your feet planted on floor and stand up quickly while raising the ball.

DOUBLE CRUNCH

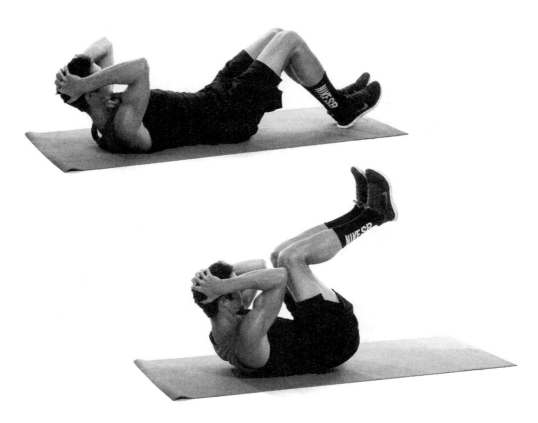

Lie on your back on the floor with your hands behind your head. Raise your legs off the floor from the hips, with your knees slightly bent. Draw your knees and your elbows toward each other by contracting the abdominal muscles. Slowly lower back to starting position, while maintaining the contraction in the abdominal muscles. Repeat 30 times.

Tip: *Try to keep the abdominal muscles contracted at all times. Be sure not to pull your neck forward with your hands; allow your abdominal muscles to do the work.*

Make It Easier: Fold your arms across your chest. Extend them in front of you to make it even easier.

SQUAT SIDEKICKS

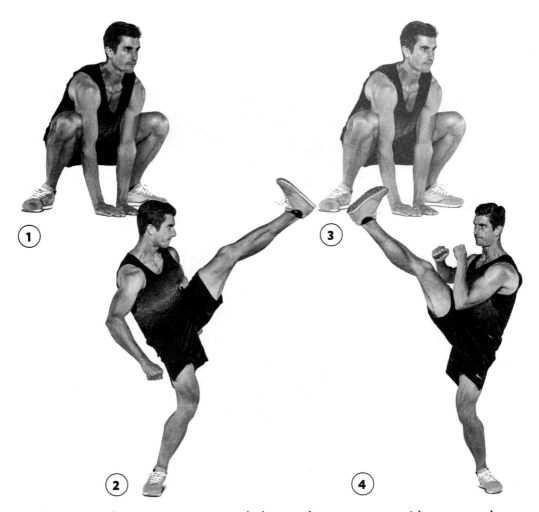

With your weight on your toes, scrunch down as low as you can, with your arms bent in front of you. Quickly stand up and pivot on your left foot, while kicking to the side with your right leg. Go back to starting position and repeat, this time kicking with your left leg. Continue alternating legs until you've performed 20 reps with each (40 total).

Works quads, glutes, hip flexors, core.

Make It Easier: Don't drop as low (just go to 90 degrees) and don't kick as high.

Make It Harder: Perform the move faster and with full range of motion.

SWOOPING COBRA PUSH-UPS

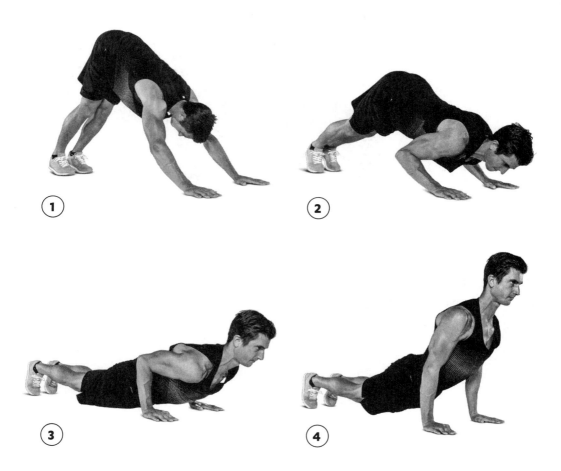

With your feet flat on the floor and your arms extended out in front of you, bend at about a 90-degree angle and place your palms on the floor. Keeping your hips high, bend your arms and swoop forward. Let your hips drop and bend your arms at 90 degrees, holding yourself off the floor. Extend your arms, lifting yourself straight up. Return to starting position. Repeat 20 times.

Make It Easier: Drop to your knees on the third movement and allow your body to rest on the floor.

PLANK

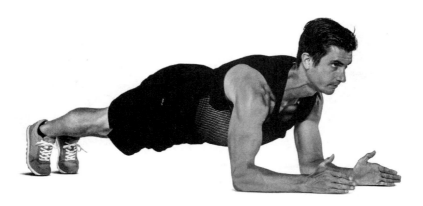

Get in the plank position, with your forearms on the floor and parallel to each other. Keep the core tight. Focusing on deep and controlled breathing, hold the plank position for 90 seconds.

RAISING VO₂ MAX

As I mentioned earlier, people with an above-average maximal oxygen consumption, or VO₂ max, have a significantly reduced risk of developing cardiovascular disease. A high VO₂ max reduces strain on the cardiovascular system during daily activities, thereby lowering physical stress. For athletes, a higher VO₂ max directly translates to improved cardiovascular efficiency and therefore performance.

Raising your VO₂ max takes under 20 minutes a week. But the training is intense, so you should attempt it only if you are in good health and have achieved a reasonable level of fitness. If you can briskly walk up four flights of stairs (two building stories) without gasping for air at the top, you are probably in good enough physical shape to begin VO₂ max training. However, just to be safe, I suggest you get a medical checkup before including VO₂ max workouts in your routine. If your health and fitness are not at a good level, work on the base Thrive Fitness program (and leave out the *VO₂ / lung power / functional strength* component) until your health and fitness have improved, and then try to boost your fitness to the next level with VO₂ max training.

The people who consistently record the highest VO₂ max are world-class cross-country skiers. However, since most of us don't have regular access to snowy backcountry trails to improve our VO₂ max, I've developed the *VO₂ / lung power / functional strength* training component that will serve this purpose and can be done pretty much anywhere.

PUTTING IT ALL TOGETHER

The basic Thrive Fitness training program can bring you many physical and non-physical benefits. However, if you combine all aspects of Thrive Fitness, you can boost your gains further, for unparalleled, sustainable benefits. Of course, this will consume more time and effort, but your return on investment will be substantial.

The complete program, which includes all fitness elements discussed in this book, will take you about 40 minutes, six days per week. Depending on your personal fitness ambitions, you may decide to pick and choose which elements to include and which to skip.

Below is a template for the six-week Thrive Fitness weight training program. I've added other activities to show how they can be worked into the program.

To summarize, VO₂ max training boosts the ability to efficiently utilize oxygen during any activity and dramatically reduces the risk of developing cardiovascular disease.

The *strength conversion / power / efficiency* workout is an efficient way to

Week #	Mon.	Tue.	Wed.	Thu.	Fri.	Sat.	Sun.
1	MBA	C	off	A	C	VLF	off
2	C	MBA	A	off	VLF	C	off
3	MBA	A	off	VLF	SPE	C	off
4	A	MBA	C	off	SPE	A	off
5	MBA	A	SPE	C	VLF	C	off
6	MBA	C	VLF	A	off	SPE	off

VLF:	VO_2 / lung power / functional strength
SPE:	Strength conversion / power / efficiency
A:	Repeat-pattern aerobic activity
MBA:	Max strength / build / afterburn
C:	Continually changing movement activity

build functional muscular strength that directly translates into fluidity of movement and reduced cardiovascular strain during daily activity. This lowers overall stress and all the symptoms related to it, greatly reduces the risk of cardiovascular and degenerative disease, and improves overall health.

Repeat-pattern aerobic activity such as a running, cycling, swimming, and rowing bolsters aerobic capacity and therefore cardiovascular fitness and health in general. It also provides non-physical benefits in the form of right-brain stimulation, which can kick-start the creative process.

Thrive Fitness *max strength / build / afterburn* workouts are performed each week of the program. This is an intense workout that builds lean muscle tissue and improves muscle strength without developing bulk. It helps dramatically improve the strength-to-weight ratio, which is a key component of any comprehensive fitness program. It also builds tendon and ligament strength and bone density.

Continually changing movement activity such as basketball, tennis, and squash augments physical brain health. Learning these new activities can help construct new neurotransmitters, which is linked to improved memory, linear thinking, and reasoning, and reduced risk of developing Alzheimer's and Parkinson's disease.

SUPERCHARGE YOUR RESULTS WITH NATURAL HUMAN GROWTH HORMONE PRODUCTION

I've come to learn that there's much more to becoming a successful athlete than simply eating and exercising—calories in, calories out. There has to be purpose with both. There also needs to be an appreciation and understanding of how training and food impact the hormonal system, and the significant value that comes with working this system to our advantage.

In my first book, *The Thrive Diet*, I write extensively about the destructive nature of chronically elevated cortisol levels, caused by stress. The first onset of elevated cortisol actually provides a surge of energy, and even increased strength. However, soon after, if cortisol becomes chronically elevated, it turns catabolic, meaning that it will eat away at muscle and cause body fat to be stored. Clearly this needs to be understood when building a program. Natural hormone manipulation can have a significant impact on results, and we can use that understanding to our advantage. Of course, we want to encourage our bodies to make less cortisol and more human growth hormone (HGH). After about the age of 30, our bodies naturally slow their production of HGH, which can lead to lean muscle loss, stored body fat, weaker bones, hair loss, reduced elasticity of skin, and other general signs of aging, including slower recovery between workouts, greater inflammation, decreased range of motion, and reduced flexibility.

natural hormone manipulation can have a significant impact on results, and we can use that understanding to our advantage

Fortunately, there are ways to help increase our HGH production, by way of properly designed workouts and well-timed, purposeful eating. The Thrive Fitness program of course takes this into consideration. Here are eight natural ways we can ensure our workout and nutrition results are maximized by boosting HGH production.

Perform VO₂ Max Training

Training above anaerobic threshold for short bursts, which engages fast-twitch muscles, helps to produce HGH. Known as VO_2 max training, this strategy is put into practice starting on page 113. Using your largest muscles, such as glutes and quads, to lift heavy weight will also release HGH. Squats and one-legged pistol squats—included in the *max strength / build / afterburn* workouts beginning on page 89—are an integral part of the hormonal manipulation utilized by Thrive Fitness.

Have a 4:1 Carbohydrate-to-Protein Ratio Recovery Drink Immediately Following a Workout

Consuming carbs on their own will cause the hormone somatostatin to be released, which directly inhibits HGH from being produced and therefore slows recovery rate. Within about 20 minutes of completing a workout, drinking a mixture that is made up of a 4:1 carb to protein ratio will help restock glycogen stores, and the protein in the mixture will prevent insulin from spiking. This will result in HGH being produced, which will significantly speed recovery by quickly bringing the body to an anabolic state. (See pages 163–166 for recovery drink recipe.)

Eat Foods That Contain Glutamine

Eating foods rich in the amino acid glutamine soon after a workout and before bed will also assist your body's HGH production. Glutamine is a nonessential amino acid, meaning the body can generate an adequate amount; however, glutamine stores become depleted when the body is under stress. Whether the stress is mental, emotional, or a result of the physical strain of exercise, glutamine levels are likely to be lower than ideal unless stress-supporting foods are a regular part of your diet. Pea protein and spinach are good sources of glutamine.

Spend Time Outside

Vitamin D that comes primarily from the sun helps the body produce more HGH. Even getting 30 minutes of sun exposure a day can have a clearly positive impact. Direct sunlight is best, but even if the sky is overcast, there's still vitamin D reaching you. Having your arms and legs exposed will turn your body into a vitamin D–harnessing machine.

Increase Melatonin Production Before Bed

Increased melatonin levels have been shown to boost HGH levels. The best way to elevate melatonin production is to limit the amount of light that enters your eyes, starting about an hour before bed. Avoiding the TV, computer, and smartphone for an hour before you go to sleep can significantly increase melatonin production, and in turn HGH production. Melatonin is naturally produced in readying your body for a deep sleep, but if there is too much light entering your eyes, its production won't ramp up.

Consume Protein Before Bed

Consuming high-quality, complete protein before bed will boost HGH. Plant-based, alkaline-forming protein in liquid form is ideal, as it's easier to digest and keeps inflammation down. Also, foods such as almonds, lentils, and pea protein have been shown to help the body naturally produce gamma-aminobutyric acid (GABA), which helps the body relax before bed and increases HGH production. (See page 182 for an HGH-releasing pre-bedtime smoothie recipe.)

Eat Foods Rich in L-arginine and L-lysine

Eating foods that are rich in the essential amino acids L-arginine and L-lysine before bed, as well as before longer, less-intense workouts, will help produce HGH. L-arginine will also enhance nitrogen oxide production, which will dilate blood vessels and therefore allow more blood to be pumped throughout your body with less strain placed on the heart. This will improve performance, as well as sleep quality, in turn allowing more HGH to be produced. Walnuts and pine nuts are an excellent source of these amino acids.

Enable Your Body to Get High-Quality Sleep

It's commonly said that we need eight hours of sleep a night to be in peak form. But I believe that quality is much more important than quantity. A person who sleeps only six hours may well be better rested than someone who sleeps a full eight, simply because the phase of the sleep is deeper. As I write about extensively in *The Thrive Diet*, reducing cortisol levels has a dramatically positive effect on enabling the body to sleep more efficiently. The deep, desirable delta phase of sleep that the body is able to reach when cortisol levels are low directly increases HGH production.

FUEL FOR FITNESS

6

EIGHT KEY NUTRIENTS

Healthy, whole food nutrition consists of many elements. The following eight are of particular value for people who are physically active.

Alkaline-Forming Foods

alkaline-forming

As I mentioned earlier, alkaline-forming foods balance the body's pH. An acidic environment adversely affects health at the cellular level; people with low body pH are therefore prone to fatigue and disease. And because acidity is a stressor, it raises cortisol levels, which results in impaired sleep quality.

To help your muscles recover and to lower your cortisol levels, consume highly alkalizing foods, such as those rich in chlorophyll, soon after exercise. Chlorophyll is the green pigment that gives leaves and green vegetables their color.

Best sources: all green vegetables, seaweed, algae (such as chlorella and spirulina)

Benefits:
Improves bone strength
Reduces inflammation
Improves muscle efficiency
Reduces risk of disease

Antioxidants

antioxidants

When our body's activity level rises, we use extra oxygen. This causes cellular oxidation, which can create free radicals. These reduce cell life span and in turn cause premature cell degeneration. Damage done by free radicals has been linked to cancer and other serious diseases and to premature skin aging. While free radicals occur naturally in the body, with small amounts being produced daily, stress can increase their presence. A reduction of stress through better nutrition combats free radical production. Antioxidants in foods help to rid the body of free radicals by escorting them out of the body.

Regular strenuous physical activity creates an abundance of free radicals. We therefore need to combat this negative side effect of exercise. Antioxidant compounds found in fruit and vegetables—vitamin C, vitamin E, selenium, and the carotenoids (compounds that give vegetables their orange color)—cancel out the effects of the cell-damaging free radicals by slowing or preventing the oxidation process. I noticed a clear improvement in how fast I recovered between workouts once I regularly began eating antioxidant-rich foods.

Best sources: berries, fruit in general, green tea

Benefits:

Protects cellular health
Speeds physical recovery
Reduces risk of disease
Improves skin appearance and
elasticity

Calcium

calcium

For most people, building, strengthening, and repairing bone is calcium's major role. Active people, however, have another important job for the mineral: muscle contraction and rhythmic heartbeat coordinator. About 95 percent of the body's calcium is stored in the skeleton, but it's the remaining few percent that is the first to decline. Calcium in the bloodstream is lost in sweat and muscle contractions, so active people need more dietary calcium. The presence of vitamin D maximizes calcium absorption. Vitamin D comes from the sun, so regular exposure to daylight will assist bone maintenance.

North Americans are developing osteoporosis and low bone density at a younger age. Initially, this was thought to be due to inadequate dietary calcium. Advertisements in magazines and on TV tried to convince people over the age of 40 to take calcium supplements. Unfortunately, the body doesn't properly absorb the inorganic forms of calcium found in supplements. So we need to consume a very large amount to have even a small impact on bone health. The net-gain principle suggests that the consumption of inorganic calcium therefore is a poor use of energy. In fact, people who take calcium supplements often suffer an energy dip soon after.

Plants take inorganic calcium from the soil and convert it into an organic form of calcium that the human body can efficiently and completely make use of. Consuming an adequate supply of organic calcium from such sources as leafy green vegetables will ensure that bones stay strong and that muscle contractions remain smooth and efficient.

We must also make sure we don't remove the calcium that already exists in our bodies. Therefore, avoid acid-forming foods, as these weaken the bones.

Best usable plant sources: dark leafy greens such as spinach, kale, collard greens; unhulled sesame seeds

Benefits:
Improves muscle function
Increases bone strength
Reduces risk of osteoporosis

Electrolytes

electrolytes

Electrolytes are electricity-conducting salts. Calcium, chloride, magnesium, potassium, and sodium are the chief electrolyte minerals. Electrolytes in body fluid and blood regulate or affect the flow of nutrients into and waste products out of cells, and are essential for muscle contractions, heartbeats, fluid regulation, and general nerve function. When too few of these minerals are ingested, we may suffer muscle cramps and heart palpitations, light-headedness and trouble concentrating. In severe cases, lack of electrolytes leads to loss of equilibrium, confusion, and inability to reason.

You may have noticed saltlike crystals forming on your face when you perspire heavily. Those are electrolytes—what's left when the water component of sweat has evaporated—and they have to be replenished through food and drink. But not just any drink. When we consume too much fluid that does not contain electrolytes, it can flush out the remaining electrolytes in our body. This is referred to as water intoxication. While it isn't common among the general population, people who perform strenuous physical activity, especially in a warm environment, are susceptible.

I have firsthand experience of water intoxication. Leading up to major races in the summer, I used to increase my water consumption considerably. One event stands out: Ironman Canada, held the last week in August in a notoriously hot part of British Columbia called the Okanagan Valley. The first couple of days, my significantly increased water consumption did not produce any noticeable adverse effects. The next couple of days, however, I became lethargic. I wasn't sure what to attribute the extra fatigue to, since I had been sleeping and eating well. Then my muscle contractions became labored. Clearly not a good development the day before a race that would involve about 9 hours of exertion in 85-degree-Fahrenheit temperatures. On race morning, as I was pulling on my wetsuit about 40 minutes before the start, my feet cramped and my legs began twitching. I got through the race, but my performance was subpar. What saved me were the sport drinks that were being handed out along the course, which contain a combination of water, sugar, and electrolytes. Had I drunk plain water, I certainly would not have been able to finish my race.

In addition to preventing cramps, proper hydration—that is, hydration with electrolytes—maintains the blood's light viscous flow, increasing the amount the heart can pump and improving performance through heartbeat efficiency and smooth, concise, yet strong muscle contractions. In the days leading up to a physically demanding event, especially if the weather is warm, sip an electrolyte drink to help improve performance. To ensure peak efficacy and improve workout quality, sip an electrolyte drink throughout the event. Continue sipping for several hours after the event is finished to improve muscle recovery.

Most commercial sport drinks contain unnecessary refined sugar and artificial flavor and color. Soon after my water intoxication ordeal, I developed my own formula for a natural, healthy, electrolyte-packed sport drink. The recipe is on page 152.

Best natural sources: coconut water, molasses and molasses sugar, seaweed (dulse and kelp in particular)

Secondary sources: bananas, tomatoes, celery

Benefits:
  Helps maintain hydration
  Improves fluidity of muscle
    contractions
  Increases the heart's efficiency, lowers
    heart rate, improves endurance
  Boosts mental clarity

Essential Fats

essential fats

Essential Fatty Acids (EFAs) are an important dietary component of overall health. The word *essential* in the name means the body cannot produce these fatty acids—they must be ingested. There are two families of EFAs: omega-3 and omega-6.

EFAs support the function of the cardiovascular, immune, and nervous systems. Responsible in part for the cells' ability to receive nutrition and eliminate waste, they play an integral role in repair and regeneration of cells, keeping the body biologically young. A balance of omega-3 and omega-6 EFAs will keep skin looking and feeling supple. EFAs also help fight infection and reduce inflammation. In addition, EFAs are linked to healthy and efficient brain development in children.

Combined with proper endurance training, a diet with an adequate supply of EFAs can help improve endurance. Our bodies can store only a small amount of muscle carbohydrate. Once the body has burned all of its carbohydrate stores, it has to be refueled—as often as every 30 minutes during a long race or workout. But after adapting to the long, slow training of Thrive Fitness, the body becomes more efficient at burning body fat as fuel and thus is able to preserve its carbohydrate stores. This means refueling doesn't have to take place as often and endurance will be significantly improved. This fuel shift is facilitated by dietary EFAs. But the fatty acids have to be properly balanced between omega-3 and omega-6.

Best sources: chia, flax, and hemp all contain a balance of both omega-3 and omega-6

Benefits:

Improves endurance
Increases the body's ability to burn body fat as fuel
Improves ability to stay well hydrated
Improves joint function

Iron

iron

Iron helps maintain the health of red blood cells so that the body can deliver oxygen-rich blood to the hardworking extremities—maximizing efficacy and therefore athletic performance. It also builds blood proteins essential for food digestion, metabolism, and circulation.

Iron is lost in sweat and is consumed during muscle contraction. The pounding impact of our feet on the ground during running can cause red blood cells to break down and thus lower their iron levels. People with low iron are at risk for anemia. Dietary iron helps counteract these problems.

About eight years ago, I went through a stage of reduced energy and poorer performance. I had a blood test to find out what was wrong. It showed that my iron level was low—not so low that

I couldn't train at all but certainly low enough to hinder my progress. I had borderline anemia. Because my active lifestyle consumed a lot of iron and because I did not eat animal products, which are higher in iron than plant-based foods, my doctor suggested I begin taking iron in tablet form. I knew a few people who had experienced stomach problems and even constipation when they began their iron supplementation program, so I wanted to see whether I could get all the iron I needed just from food. I found that there are many good plant-based sources of iron.

Best plant-based sources: pumpkin seeds, leafy greens (especially kale). Vega One contains 100 percent of the recommended daily allowance.

Benefits:
> Improves blood's oxygen-carrying ability
> Increases physical stamina
> Boosts energy

Phytonutrients

phytonutrients

Phytonutrients are plant compounds that offer health benefits independent of their nutritional value. They are not essential for life, but they can help improve vitality and quality of life.

For example, a phytonutrient found in tomatoes improves blood vessel elasticity and thereby enhances blood flow through the heart. Tomatoes can thus help reduce the risk of developing cardiovascular disease and enhance athletic performance. The heavy processing of fruit and vegetables will reduce the amount and effectiveness of phytonutrients, so they are best eaten raw. Every type of fruit and vegetable has at least a few phytonutrients, so simply eating many servings on a daily basis will boost health and therefore performance.

Turmeric and chia contain inflammation-reducing phytonutrients. When eaten after exercise, they reduce aches and pains and speed recovery. They may also reduce the risk of developing arthritis and Alzheimer's. Some people dislike the taste of turmeric, so I have listed it as optional in the recipes.

Best sources: vegetables, chia, turmeric

Benefits:
> Improves heart health
> Reduces risk of cardiovascular disease
> Improves blood vessel elasticity, thereby improving circulation

Raw Food

raw

As I noted earlier, eating a large percentage of raw food makes sense on several levels. High-temperature cooking and processing of food destroys enzymes and nutrients needed for efficient digestion. Before the body can make use of cooked food, it must produce enzymes to aid in the digestion process. That takes work, which of course is an energy draw and therefore creates a nominal amount of stress. In addition, food containing both sugar and fat cooked at a high temperature can provoke an immune response that causes inflammation.

Best plant-based sources: fruit, nuts, seeds, and most vegetables. Vegetables that contain a high amount of starch such as potatoes and sweet potatoes are best eaten cooked and only occasionally.

Benefits:

Improves digestibility of most foods
Maintains higher nutritional value in most foods
Provides higher net gain, more energy

TOP FOODS FOR PEAK PERFORMANCE

With the information on nutrition gained during my racing career, and some additional research, I compiled a list of top foods that offer a robust combination of all eight dietary components listed above. These foods boost athletic and mental performance and are particularly beneficial to people who are physically active and lead a fast-paced life. A few years after I began racing, I *based* my diet on—not just *supplemented* it with—these foods. Since then, I've worked with several top professional athletes in a variety of sports, both strength and endurance, and have found these foods to offer significant benefit.

Beginning on page 149 are 33 recipes, 21 of which are sport-specific recipes made from this set of core ingredients. More recipes are available in *The Thrive Diet*, *Whole Foods to Thrive*, and *Thrive Energy Cookbook*.

As indicated by the icons, these foods are particularly high in several of the eight key nutritional components and thus complement and advance the progress of the Thrive Fitness exercise program.

Açaí Berries

antioxidants   electrolytes   essential fats   phytonutrients   raw

Açaí berries are the small, purple fruit of palm trees that grow in marshy areas in Central and South America, where the fruit has been eaten by native peoples for centuries.

The berries are exceptionally rich in antioxidants and contain essential fatty acids and amino acids. Because they are also easy to digest, açaí are a high net-gain food that can speed recovery after exercise.

In North America, açaí can be bought in most health food stores either frozen whole or freeze-dried in powdered form. The frozen berries are handy for making a smoothie. And you can mix the powder into recipes such as energy bars for an easy way to boost nutritional content.

Agave Nectar

phytonutrients   raw

Like all fruit, agave nectar is easily digested, but because of its high fructose content, it has a slower release of complex carbohydrates. Especially useful as fuel for athletic performance, agave nectar has a honeylike consistency and a light, sweet taste that makes it easy and pleasant to ingest while exercising. The high fructose of agave nectar is an ideal complement to the high glucose found in dates. I use agave nectar combined with dates in several of my sport-specific recipes. It is also a good choice for a healthy sweetener; it can be used in place of honey or sugar in many conventional recipes.

Buckwheat

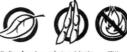

alkaline-forming phytonutrients   raw

Buckwheat is not actually wheat; it is a seed in the rhubarb family. Containing eight essential amino acids, including quite high amounts of the often-elusive tryptophan, buckwheat is a good source of protein. Tryptophan is a precursor to the neurotransmitter serotonin; having an adequate amount of tryptophan in the diet can be important to help enhance mood and mental clarity. Buckwheat is also high in vitamins E and B, calcium, and especially manganese.

Since buckwheat is gluten-free, it is considerably more alkaline-forming than gluten-containing grains. It is also a slow-release carbohydrate. Combined with a simple carbohydrate, buckwheat becomes one of the best endurance fuels available. Sprouted buckwheat digests and burns even more effectively because the sprouting process converts the complex carbohydrate into sugar, which the body can burn more efficiently than starch. But since the protein, fat, and fiber remain, this sugar will not cause an insulin spike and subsequent crash.

I use buckwheat groats, the hulled seeds of the buckwheat plant, as the base ingredient for my pre- and post-workout drinks. Recipes start on page 151.

Chia

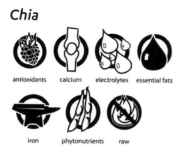

antioxidants   calcium   electrolytes   essential fats

iron   phytonutrients   raw

Chia seeds are small and round, and they look like poppy seeds (there are white chia seeds as well). Grown in the Amazon basin in Peru, and now cultivated in other parts of the world such as Australia, chia laps up the nutrients in the rich, fertile soil and passes them on to the consumer. With a unique crunchy texture, chia is gaining in popularity in North America.

Particularly high in magnesium, potassium, calcium, and iron, chia can effectively replenish minerals used in muscle contractions and lost in sweat. Chia is truly one of the top foods for active people. And because it is high in both soluble and insoluble fiber, which helps to sustain energy and maintain fullness, chia is a true high net-gain food. Packed with antioxidants and containing about 20 percent high-quality protein, chia is an ideal food to help speed recovery after exercise.

Aztec warriors were rumored to eat chia before going into battle to give them a nutritional boost and thereby improve their endurance. They were also said to have carried it with them when they ran long distances to be used as their body's primary fuel source. Since chia is nutritionally well rounded and complete, this may well have been the case.

I mix ground chia seeds into my pre- and post-exercise drinks (recipes start on page 156). I also include them in my energy gel recipes (starting on page 153). Chia seeds are ideal to help maintain energy level during a workout and are remarkably easy to digest.

Chlorella

alkaline-forming   antioxidants   essential fats   phytonutrients   raw

Nutritionally speaking, the green algae chlorella is a true superfood, containing 65 percent protein; essential fatty acids; and a plethora of vitamins, minerals, and enzymes. Chlorella contains vitamin B12, which is extremely hard for vegetarians and vegans to find in forms other than laboratory-created tablets. Chlorella also possesses all 10 of the essential amino acids—the ones that must be obtained through diet. The amino acids present, in conjunction with naturally occurring enzymes, are the most easily absorbed and utilized form of protein available. Many other complete proteins are much more energy-intensive to digest; by comparison, chlorella is a particularly high net-gain food.

Coconut Oil

raw

Coconut oil, produced by pressing the meat of the coconut, thereby removing the fiber, is one of the top fuel sources for active people. It is exceptionally easy to digest and provides quick and sustained energy that burns efficiently. Unlike other vegetable oils, which remain liquid unless stored at low temperatures, coconut oil turns solid below 75 degrees Fahrenheit.

Coconut oil is a form of saturated fat but, in contrast to most saturated fats, it is good for you. Unlike regular saturated fat, which is stored in the cells, this fat is utilized in the liver, where it is converted to energy closely resembling glucose. Because it burns efficiently, this fat is much easier on the pancreas, liver, and digestive system than are standard fats. Coconut oil is becoming the fat of choice for those intent on achieving or maintaining a lean body.

I use coconut oil in some of my energy bar recipes (starting on page 167), as well as in the next-generation energy gel recipes (starting on page 153).

Coconut Water

electrolytes   raw

Coconut water is the nearly translucent fluid inside the coconut (not to be confused with coconut milk, which is a combination of coconut water blended with coconut meat). It has a light, sweet flavor. It is fat-free and contains high levels of simple carbohydrates, making it an ideal fluid to boost muscle glycogen without causing the stomach to become bogged down with digestive duties.

Packed with electrolytes, coconut water is the original sport drink. It has been used for decades to properly hydrate people who sweat profusely in tropical regions. I use coconut water as the base ingredient for several of my sport drink recipes, starting on page 151. Be sure to look for pure coconut water, with no additional sugars or flavors.

Dates

raw

Dates are nearly pure glucose, which, in its natural form, is a valuable type of sugar for people who are active. Glucose is rapidly converted to glycogen in the liver. Maintaining an adequate glycogen supply in both the muscles and the liver is imperative for sustained energy. For that reason, dates are best consumed shortly before, during, or immediately following exercise. Chlorophyll-rich foods also convert to glycogen, but not as quickly as glucose, therefore making the easily digestible, alkaline-forming date the ideal snack to fuel activity.

I use dates as the base ingredient for my whole food energy bar recipes, starting on page 168.

Flaxseed

essential fats   phytonutrients   raw

Grown mostly in the Canadian prairies, the seed of the blue-flowering flax plant is prized for its lignans and high omega-3 fatty acid content. The regular inclusion of lignans in the diet has been shown to reduce the risk of cancer. Flaxseed is also rich in fiber. However, it is the omega-3 EFA content that makes flaxseed most valuable to athletes. As I noted earlier, aside from its ability to help reduce inflammation caused by movement, omega-3 plays an integral part in the metabolism of fat. A diet with a daily dose of 1 tablespoon of whole flaxseed will allow the body to more efficiently burn body fat as fuel. This is obviously a benefit to anyone wanting to shed body fat, but it is of major im-

portance to athletes, who need to spare the energy stored in the muscles. As the body becomes proficient at burning fat as fuel (by training and proper diet), endurance significantly improves.

Whole flaxseed is high in potassium, an electrolyte responsible in part for smooth muscle contractions. Potassium is lost in sweat, so it must be replaced regularly to keep the body's levels adequately stocked. Potassium also helps to maintain fluid balance, assisting with the hydration process. Flaxseed is a whole food and a complete protein, and retains its enzymes, allowing it to be absorbed and utilized by the body with ease, improving immune function.

Greens

alkaline-forming   calcium   iron   phytonutrients   raw

Because of their chlorophyll content, green foods are an excellent way to help alkalize the body, which, as I mentioned before, reduces inflammation and helps maintain bone health.

Chlorophyll also cleanses and oxygenates the blood, making it a true performance enhancer. More available oxygen in the blood translates to better endurance and an overall reduction in fatigue. In their raw state, chlorophyll-containing plants also possess an abundance of live enzymes that promote the quick rejuvenation of our cells. The consumption of green foods after exercise has been shown to help speed cellular regeneration. The consumption of chlorophyll-rich, leafy green vegetables combined with moderate exercise is the best way to create a biologically younger body. Ounce for ounce, dark greens are also an excellent source of iron and calcium.

You may not crave a plate full of fibrous, leafy green vegetables immediately after exercise, and they'd take up room in your stomach needed for other post-recovery nutrition. An easy way to ingest greens immediately after exercise is to mix a greens powder such as chlorella or spirulina into a fruit-based post-exercise recovery drink. Recipes start on page 165. Later in the day, a big salad is ideal.

Green Tea

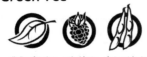

alkaline-forming   antioxidants   phytonutrients

While green, or incompletely fermented, tea leaves do contain a form of caffeine, it differs significantly from the form found in coffee beans. This form of caffeine, called theophylline, causes a slow, steady release of energy over the course of several hours. Therefore, it does not cause caffeine jitters and places less stress on the adrenal glands.

Green tea is also rich in chlorophyll and antioxidants.

However, since green tea is classified as a stimulant, it is something that I suggest drinking only before physical exercise. Green tea can help improve the level of intensity a person can reach during a workout or on race day. This leads to better, faster results. Theophylline has also been shown to help improve focus and concentration and to calm nerves. Before a big race, being able to relax and focus are valuable traits. I use steeped green tea in my pre-workout drinks; recipes start on page 157.

Hemp

alkaline-forming   antioxidants   essential fats   phytonutrients   raw

Hemp is available in three basic forms: seed, powder, and oil. Hemp seeds come straight from the plant and are rich in omega-3 and omega-6 essential fatty acids. When pressed, the seed becomes hemp powder and oil. The powder, sometimes referred to as flour, is then milled finer to remove some of the starch. The result is hemp protein.

The protein present in hemp is complete, containing all 10 essential amino acids, which boosts the immune system and hastens recovery. Hemp foods also have natural anti-inflammatory properties, key factors for speeding the repair of soft tissue damage caused by physical activity. Raw hemp products maintain their naturally high level of vitamins, minerals, high-quality balanced fats, antioxidants, fiber, and the very alkaline chlorophyll. Edestin, an amino acid present only in hemp, is considered an integral part of DNA. It makes hemp the closest plant source to our own human amino acid profile.

When it comes to protein, quality, not quantity, is paramount. I find hemp protein the easiest protein to digest. Since it is raw, its naturally occurring digestive enzymes remain intact. That and its relatively high pH allow it to be easily used by the body. As a result, the digestive strain placed on the body to absorb and utilize protein is reduced. High-quality, complete protein such as hemp is instrumental not only to muscle tissue regeneration, but also to fat metabolism. Protein ingestion instigates the release of a hormone that enables the body to more easily utilize its fat reserves, thereby improving endurance and facilitating body fat loss.

Maca

phytonutrients

Maca, a root vegetable with medicinal qualities, is native to the high Andes of Bolivia and Peru. Known as an adaptogen, maca curtails the effects of stress by aiding the regeneration of the adrenal glands, making it an ideal food for the modern world. It helps lower cortisol levels, which will improve sleep quality. Of course, better-quality sleep directly translates into more waking energy. And maca increases energy by means of nourishment, not stimulation. I have found that I am better able to adapt to physical stress when I add maca to my diet.

Maca is a rich source of steroidlike compounds found in both plants and animals that promote quick regeneration of fatigued muscle tissue. During the off-season, I make a concerted effort to build strength and muscle mass in the gym. I've experienced exceptional strength gains by adding maca to my recovery drink. I can lift more weight than in previous years and I recover faster. It has enabled me to perform more high-quality workouts, thereby advancing my progress.

Published human clinical studies of maca used the gelatinized form of the vegetable. Gelatinization removes the hard-to-digest starchy component of the maca root. The result is an easily digestible, quickly assimilated, and more concentrated form of maca. Gelatinized maca has a pleasant, nutty taste and dissolves more easily than regular maca. When selecting maca, be sure to choose the gelatinized form for best results.

Sea Vegetables

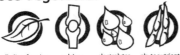

alkaline-forming   calcium   electrolytes   phytonutrients   raw

Packed with nutrients, sea vegetables are among the most nutritionally dense foods available. Containing about 10 times the calcium of cow's milk and several times more iron than red meat, sea vegetables deliver nutrition in an easily digestible, alkaline-forming package.

Sea vegetables are the richest known source of naturally occurring electrolytes. They are also full of chlorophyll and easy to digest. Dulse, nori, and kelp are the best-known sea vegetables in North America.

To maintain hydration during physical activity, I found it helpful to drink a sport drink containing a small amount of sea vegetables. Since there was no such sport drink on the market, I made my own (recipe on page 152).

Yerba Maté

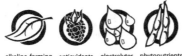

alkaline-forming   antioxidants   electrolytes   phytonutrients

Yerba maté is a species of holly native to subtropical South America. The leaves are rich in chlorophyll, antioxidants, and numerous trace minerals and help aid digestion. However, since yerba maté does contain a form of caffeine, I suggest drinking it in a similar fashion to green tea: before exercise or when you really need extra short-term energy. Yerba maté is one of the healthiest forms of stimulation, yet any kind of stimulation will take its toll on the adrenal glands eventually.

I use yerba maté in several of my pre-workout drinks (recipes for sport drinks start on page 158). However, after drinking yerba maté, it's important to make sure the adrenals are well nourished to help speed recovery. I include maca in my post-workout drink for this reason.

When buying yerba maté, avoid products from plantation-style farms that have cleared old-growth forest. Be sure to choose a brand that is wild harvest or has been grown with the jungle, not instead of the jungle. By making the harvesting of wild yerba maté economically viable for the producers, you will help prevent clearance of old-growth rain forest for the farming of animals. Before yerba maté rose to popularity outside of South America, it was common for large plots of land to be clear-cut for cattle-grazing land. While this is still a problem, those areas that have an abundance of yerba maté growing within the jungle can be harvested without any alteration to the forest canopy; therefore, the value of the natural foliage is greater, in many cases, than cattle pasture, so it will be preserved.

PERFORMANCE FUEL FOR PRE- AND POST-WORKOUT

For many years, athletes have been told to consume copious amounts of complex carbohydrate. Since sugar burns rapidly and fiber has little effect on blood sugar, the starch component of carbohydrate (also known as complex carbohydrate) was emphasized for a fuel source. Starch-rich foods include pasta, wheat flour, and potatoes.

While complex carbohydrates release energy at a slower rate than simple carbohydrates and therefore will not cause a sharp blood sugar crash, they have a commonly overlooked fault. What complex carbohydrates make up for in sustained energy release, they lose in digestibility and efficient transfer from food into energy. In addition, refined, processed complex carbohydrates such as those found in regular pasta and white bread cause inflammation. Having an exceptionally low pH and therefore a significantly acid-forming attribute, refined foods will promote inflammation and therefore reduce performance by hampering efficiency.

In contrast, carbohydrate in raw fruit and sprouted buckwheat, for example, helps reduce inflammation, leading to quicker recovery from exercise, better joint mobility, and therefore improved endurance.

When I first started training for endurance, I followed the advice of conventional sport nutrition books and ate enormous amounts of complex carbohydrates. But I found that loading up on pasta, bread, and potatoes caused my energy level to drop. And I didn't notice any improvement in endurance. It wasn't until later that I discovered how to truly boost pre-workout and race performance through non-starchy whole foods such as fruit and sprouted seeds.

Pre-Workout Fuel

As you will notice from the sample menu plan (see page 183), I suggest consuming an easily digestible form of carbohydrate before each workout as a means of raising blood sugar. The best sources of simple carbohydrates such as glucose and fructose are fruit and sprouted seeds. When seeds are sprouted, their starch component converts to sugar. The body cannot make use of starch without first converting it into sugar. The sprouting process does it for us, saving our body energy and significantly improving ability. Sprouted buckwheat is a particularly good whole food fuel for peak athletic performance.

When fueling up for longer workouts, make sure to consume a small amount of protein, soluble fiber, and fat (such as hemp, pea protein, pumpkin seed, chia, flaxseed). This will help slow the rate at which carbohydrate will be released into the bloodstream, thereby allowing its energy to be spread over a longer period of time. Simply put, this approach will increase endurance.

Sprouted buckwheat contains about 20 percent protein and a small amount of soluble fiber for staying power. Dates supply the simple carbohydrate for an ideal pre-workout formula. The ideal ratio of carbohydrate to protein to ensure optimal energy release for a longer workout is about 3:1. Meaning that the pre-workout snack should contain three grams of carbohydrate for every gram of protein. I have developed a pre-workout snack that provides that ratio in an easily digestible form. The recipes begin on page 168.

The figures below and on the next page illustrate how simple carbohydrates enter the bloodstream quickly, give a short burst of energy, and then drop quickly after about 10 minutes, at which point refueling is necessary to maintain high-level exercise. When simple carbohydrates are ingested together with protein, soluble fiber, and fat, the spike is significantly less pronounced. The energy level is more constant and endurance is improved. Depending on the fitness level (and therefore the efficiency) of the athlete, refueling won't be required until about 45 minutes to 2 hours later.

In addition to ensuring steady energy release, there are a few other measures we can take to improve workout quality. Within about two hours leading up to a longer workout or race, most people, myself included, prefer not to eat due to the high probability of stomach upset. The anxiety that sometimes accompanies the hours before a race can also adversely affect the efficacy of the digestion

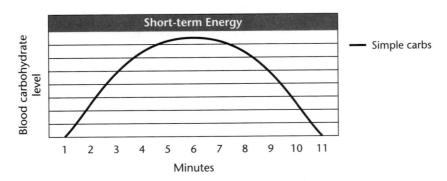

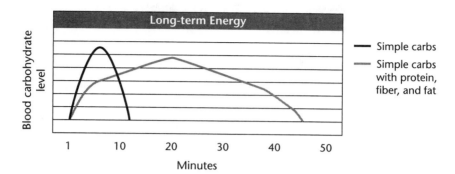

process. Then there's the physical activity itself. We want to avoid requiring the stomach to draw upon extra blood to aid digestion. During exercise, blood is needed in the extremities to deliver oxygen and remove waste products; requiring it to also be at work in the stomach will reduce endurance. In addition, too much food in the stomach is the leading cause of painful diaphragm stitch. In light of this, I have formulated the pre-workout drink to digest easily while providing energy immediately before activity. Recipes start on page 157.

Post-Workout Nutrition

The nutritional aspects of the post-workout snack should, in many cases, mirror those of the pre-workout snack. First, it will need to be easy to digest. Post-exertion, blood needs to be circulating in the extremities to deliver nutrition to all the cells in an attempt to begin the recovery process. If we eat a heavy meal that requires extra blood for digestion, we reduce the amount of blood that can flow freely in the rest of the body.

The sources of carbohydrate will also be the same: one that contains sugar in the form of quick-acting glucose, and another with slower release carbohydrates, combined with protein, insoluble fiber, and fat. However, the ratio of carbohydrate to protein will need to be 4:1 instead of 3:1.

Longer and harder training sessions deplete the adrenals, so I add maca to my post-workout drink to help the adrenals make a quick recovery. And "borrowed" energy from the pre-workout drink in the form of green tea and yerba maté needs to be paid back to prevent adrenal fatigue later in the week.

33 THRIVE
PERFORMANCE RECIPES

7

The following whole food sport-specific recipes are ones I've made for several years to help raise performance while avoiding common less-healthy store-bought options. Each ingredient in every recipe has a specific purpose: whether it's muscle-fueling carbohydrates, energy-prolonging electrolytes, or easily digestible proteins. I've included a few of my favorite non-sport recipes as well. They help supply balanced nutrients that fuel muscles as well as facilitate their ongoing growth and repair.

Whenever making recipes from whole foods, it can be difficult to get the measurements exactly right each time. A fluctuation in temperature and moisture level during the growing season can have a noticeable impact on the moisture level of the ingredient. Another factor that can affect moisture content is the transportation and storage of ingredients. This being the case, if a recipe

seems too dry, simply add more of a wet ingredient. And if too much moisture is present, add more of a dry ingredient to balance it.

SPORT-SPECIFIC RECIPES

Although it seems logical that athletes would eat, or at least want to eat, top-quality food, until recently, athletes have been content to fuel themselves with highly refined and processed "energy" foods. At first I thought this was primarily a result of the slick marketing and large promotional budgets of the major players in the industry. But it became strikingly apparent to me that many in the athletic community as a whole did not appreciate the far-reaching effects of high-quality performance foods. I'm not exaggerating when I say that it's not uncommon for athletes to actually eat worse than the regular population.

But athletes are not immune to the effects of poor-quality food. True, if we make poor dietary choices, we don't develop excess body fat or other visual signs of poor nutrition as quickly as our sedentary counterparts. But the long-term shortcomings of poor nutrition will be magnified. People who exercise regularly break down cellular tissue during every workout. Food serves as the building blocks of reconstruction. And we all know that poor-quality construction materials result in a poor-quality structure. *Filler cells* is the term used for body tissue reconstructed by means of refined, low-grade, nutrient-absent food and foodlike substances. If body reconstruction with filler cells continues, the body degenerates. This is the first significant stage of premature aging. Next comes the looser skin, slowed recovery after exercise, reduced flexibility and mobility, joint pain, and generalized aches. As we now know, the signs of aging aren't necessarily related to our age in years; they are related to our biological age.

However, I'm pleased to say that this antiquated way of viewing exercise and nutrition is much less prevalent. Still, I was simply not able to find commercial versions of sport-specific products that I felt would be a wise biological investment. For years I used to eat the stan-dard commercial bars before a race. While they put an end to my immediate hunger, I never felt as though they digested efficiently. I would often get an upset stomach moments before or during the race. And the energy they provided was short-lived. Necessity motivated me to create a fuel that digested easily and provided sustained energy—a homemade, sport-specific line of whole foods. So I decided to implement what I had learned about whole food nutrition and its substantial contribution to overall health and performance gains by creating some recipes.

Each of the following recipes can play an integral role in the athlete's overall nutrition program and success. They are made with natural, plant-based, nutrient-dense, easy-to-digest (and therefore exceptionally high net-gain) whole food sources that are synergistically combined for a specific function. Over the years, the recipes have evolved into what I consider to be among the best fuel and building blocks for active people. I include the recipes for the whole line below. Soon after I began writing this book, I decided to make a commercial version of this sport line. It is called Vega Sport. Details begin on page 186.

Note: Each drink recipe makes about 1 large serving or 2 small servings.

Basic Electrolyte Energy Drink

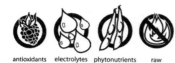

antioxidants   electrolytes   phytonutrients   raw

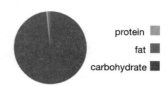

protein
fat
carbohydrate

I often make this simple drink the night before a race or major workout, and sip it throughout the following morning to be properly hydrated and to get energized and focused for the task ahead. Since yerba maté is a stimulant, be sure to have a recovery drink after the workout or race that includes maca, to help rebuild the adrenal glands. Recipes for recovery drinks start on page 163.

1½ cups coconut water
1 yerba maté tea bag (or substitute 1 tsp loose yerba maté)

Pour the coconut water into a cup. Add the yerba maté and let steep overnight at room temperate or in the fridge (this drink tastes much better cold). There's no need for heat if you let it steep overnight.

Classic Lemon Lime Sport Drink

antioxidants   electrolytes   phytonutrients   raw

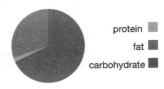

protein
fat
carbohydrate

Dates are high in glucose, which will enter the bloodstream almost instantly. The sugar in the coconut water will enter the bloodstream more slowly, spreading out the energy over a longer period.

2 large Medjool dates
2 cups coconut water
1 tsp coconut oil
Juice from ½ lemon
Juice from ¼ lime
Sea salt to taste
1 tsp dried dulse flakes (optional)

If you prefer your drink smooth, strain out any pulp from the lemon and lime juice. Blend all the ingredients together in a blender. Add 1 tsp dried dulse flakes to boost electrolytes.

Next-Generation Energy Gels

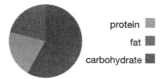

protein ▨
fat ▨
carbohydrate ▨

The energy gel recipes in *The Thrive Diet* work well, but these are even better. These contain coconut oil, which provides direct energy to the liver and dramatically improves endurance when combined with a carbohydrate source.

And these contain chia, which provides sustained nutrients in an easily digestible whole food form. When the energy from the glucose contained in the dates begins to wear off, the slower-release energy from the chia and agave nectar kicks in.

The gels can be put in a small, resealable plastic bag and carried on long workouts or during a race. However, they are easier to handle and consume when carried in a gel flask. These can be bought at most running stores.

Cacao Energy Gel

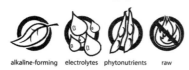

alkaline-forming   electrolytes   phytonutrients   raw

2 large Medjool dates
1 tbsp agave nectar
1 tbsp ground chia
1 tbsp coconut oil
1 tsp lemon zest
1 tbsp fresh lemon juice
1 tsp cacao nibs (or substitute carob powder)
Sea salt to taste
1 tsp ground yerba maté (optional)

Blend all the ingredients together in a blender to a gel-like consistency. For an extra kick, add 1 tsp ground yerba maté.

Orange Energy Gel

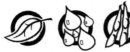

alkaline-forming　electrolytes　phytonutrients　raw

2 large Medjool dates
1 tbsp agave nectar
1 tbsp ground chia
1 tbsp coconut oil
½ tbsp orange zest
½ tsp dulse
Sea salt to taste
1 tsp ground yerba maté (optional)

Blend all the ingredients together in a blender to a gel-like consistency. For an extra kick, add 1 tsp ground yerba maté.

Chocolate Vega Energy Pudding

antioxidants   calcium   essential fats   iron   phytonutrients

A nutritionally balanced blend of easily digestible, high-nutrient foods, this pudding is an ideal pre-exercise snack. Or serve it as a high-energy mid-afternoon boost.

2 bananas
1 cup blueberries
2 scoops Chocolate Vega One
¼ cup soaked raw almonds or almond butter
1 tbsp coconut oil
1 tsp fresh lemon juice
¼ tsp sea salt
2 tbsp chia or hemp seeds (optional)

Process everything in a food processor until smooth and creamy. For extra flavor, texture, and nutrition, add a couple of tablespoons of chia or hemp seeds.

MAKES 2 SERVINGS.

Pre-Long Workout or Race Drinks

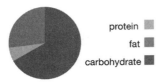

protein
fat
carbohydrate

To provide staying power, the optimal carbohydrate to protein ratio immediately before a longer workout or race is about three parts carbohydrate to one part protein. The pre-workout drinks also contain a healthy form of caffeine from green tea and yerba maté to improve endurance in an athletic event. They are both good sources of antioxidants. Green tea is particularly good at calming nerves and allowing the mind to stay focused. Yerba maté is loaded with trace minerals and can boost energy levels for the duration of a workout. However, since they are also both stimulants, a nutrient-rich recovery drink that contains maca to help the adrenals recover will be an important part of the recovery process. Recipes for such drinks begin on pages 163 and 180.

These drinks digest easily and are packed with energy-producing nutrients and fuel. I am sure you will notice performance gains once you start including these drinks. In particularly hot conditions, consider substituting half the water with coconut water to boost electrolyte content. An excellent alternative to these drinks is 1 scoop of Vega One (or 3 scoops of Vega Protein and Greens) blended with ½ cup of berries and 1 banana (to make the carbohydrate to protein ratio about 3:1) and about 1½ cups of water. To make with green tea or yerba maté, simply brew and use in place of water.

Each recipe makes 1 large serving or 2 small servings. The amount you drink depends on your appetite.

Pre-covery HGH-Releasing Smoothie

alkaline-forming   antioxidants   essential fats   iron   phytonutrients

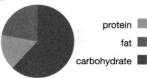

protein
fat
carbohydrate

This is an antioxidant-rich pre-longer-workout smoothie (run more than 90 minutes, bike more than 120 minutes, etc., repeat pattern). The antioxidants from the blackberries and blueberries ensure that free radical damage is kept to a minimum (I call it pre-covery), and the walnuts and pine nuts supply L-arginine and L-lysine, which will encourage HGH production during longer, less intense workouts. This will reduce muscles catabolization and enhance body fat burn rate.

1 cup blueberries
½ cup blackberries
¼ cup walnuts
¼ cup pine nuts
1½ cups water (1 cup if you prefer it to be thicker;
    or substitute brewed green tea)
1 tsp fresh lemon juice
1 tsp greens powder (chlorella or spirulina)
1 scoop Vega Sport Performance Protein (or pea protein)

Blend all ingredients together in a blender.

Long-Lasting Lemon Lime Drink

alkaline-forming   electrolytes   phytonutrients   raw

1 yerba maté tea bag
1 green tea tea bag
2 cups water (for steeping)
3 large Medjool dates
1 tbsp coconut oil
1 tbsp hemp protein
1 tbsp ground chia
1 tbsp sprouted buckwheat groats (or substitute cooked)
Juice from ½ lemon
Juice from ¼ lime
½ tsp lemon zest

The night before your event or a particularly hard workout, brew 1 cup of yerba maté and 1 cup of green tea. Let steep for about 10 minutes, remove the tea bags, and put the cups with tea in the fridge. When you're ready for your drink, blend the teas and the remaining ingredients together in a blender.

Blueberry Smoothie

alkaline-forming antioxidants electrolytes phytonutrients raw

1 yerba maté tea bag
1 green tea tea bag
2 cups water (for steeping)
2 large Medjool dates
½ cup blueberries
1 tbsp coconut oil
1 tbsp hemp protein
1 tbsp ground chia
1 tbsp sprouted buckwheat groats (or substitute cooked)
Juice from ½ lemon
Juice from ¼ lime
½ tsp lemon zest

Brew 1 cup of yerba maté and 1 cup of green tea. Discard the tea bags and blend all the ingredients together in a blender. If you don't mind a slightly gritty consistency, instead of brewing, blend loose yerba maté, loose green tea, and the water with the other ingredients.

Chocolate Smoothie

alkaline-forming   electrolytes   phytonutrients   raw

1 yerba maté tea bag
1 green tea tea bag
2 cups water (for steeping)
3 large Medjool dates
1 tbsp coconut oil
1 tbsp hemp protein
1 tbsp ground chia
1 tbsp sprouted buckwheat grouts (or substitute cooked)
Juice from ½ lemon
1 tbsp raw carob (or substitute roasted)

Brew 1 cup of yerba maté and 1 cup of green tea. Discard the tea bags and blend all the ingredients together in a blender. If you don't mind a slightly gritty consistency, instead of brewing, blend loose yerba maté, loose green tea, and the water with the other ingredients.

Papaya Ginger Smoothie

alkaline-forming   electrolytes   phytonutrients   raw

1 yerba maté tea bag
1 green tea tea bag
2 cups water (for steeping)
2 large Medjool dates
½ cup chopped fresh papaya
1 tbsp coconut oil
1 tbsp hemp protein
1 tbsp ground chia
1 tbsp sprouted buckwheat groats (or substitute cooked)
Juice from ½ lemon
Juice from ¼ lime
1 tsp grated fresh ginger

Brew 1 cup of yerba maté and 1 cup of green tea. Discard the tea bags and blend all the ingredients together in a blender. If you don't mind a slightly gritty consistency, instead of brewing, blend loose yerba maté, loose green tea, and the water with the other ingredients.

Long Workout or Race Recovery Drinks

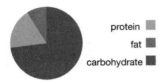

protein
fat
carbohydrate

After a particularly draining workout, one that has depleted glycogen stores, these recovery drinks are ideal to replenish and rebuild. After a run that lasts longer than an hour, a particularly hard weight training session, or any activity that is beyond what your body is accustomed to, you need to ingest the correct ratio of carbohydrate to protein to help speed recovery. The ideal ratio is four grams of carbohydrate for every gram of protein. These recovery drinks therefore have more protein than the sport drinks and gels but less than the pre-workout drinks. Have a recovery drink within 20 minutes of completing your exercise session. A few hours later, drink a regular smoothie, which contains more protein, to continue the recovery process. An excellent alternative to these recovery drinks is 1 scoop of Vega One blended with 1 cup of berries and 1 banana (to make the carbohydrate to protein ratio about 4:1), about 1 cup of water, and 1 cup of coconut water.

Each recipe makes about 1 large serving or 2 small servings. The amount you drink depends on your appetite.

Cookies and Cream Recovery Smoothie

(From *Thrive Energy Cookbook*)

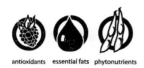

antioxidants   essential fats   phytonutrients

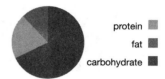

protein
fat
carbohydrate

Ideal for strength athletes in pursuit of building lean mass, this recovery smoothie is a delicious way to feed your fatigued muscles while reducing inflammation and oxidative damage to your cells. Popularized at the Thrive Energy Lab by those who just spent themselves at the gym.

2 tbsp raw cashews
2 tbsp vegan dark chocolate chips
1 tbsp cacao nibs
1 tbsp raw cashew butter
1 tbsp pitted and chopped Medjool dates
1 scoop vanilla Vega Sport Performance Protein
1 cup unsweetened almond milk
¼ cup agave nectar or maple syrup (optional)
About 2 cups ice

In a blender, combine all the ingredients except the ice. Add ice to about 1 inch above the liquid line. Blend on high speed until smooth and creamy.

The optional agave is suggested if your workout has exceeded 90 minutes.

Carob Mint Recovery Drink

alkaline-forming   calcium   electrolytes   phytonutrients   raw

4 large Medjool dates
2 cups water
1 tbsp hemp protein
1 tbsp ground chia
2 tbsp sprouted buckwheat groats (or substitute cooked)
1 tbsp raw carob (or substitute roasted)
1 tsp ground dulse flakes
1 tsp maca
1 tsp greens powder (chlorella or spirulina)
1 tbsp fresh mint

Blend all the ingredients together in a blender.

Chocolate Vega Recovery Drink

alkaline-forming   antioxidants   calcium   electrolytes   essential fats   iron   phytonutrients

1 large Medjool date
¾ cup chopped fresh pineapple
1 cup water
1 cup coconut water
1 tbsp sprouted buckwheat groats (or substitute cooked)
1 medium banana
1 scoop Chocolate Vega One

Blend all the ingredients together in a blender.

Lemon Lime Recovery Drink

alkaline-forming   calcium   electrolytes   phytonutrients   raw

4 large Medjool dates
2 cups water
1 tbsp hemp protein
1 tbsp ground chia
2 tbsp sprouted buckwheat groats (or substitute cooked)
Juice from ½ lemon
Juice from ¼ lime
½ tsp lemon zest
1 tsp ground dulse flakes
1 tsp maca
1 tsp greens powder (chlorella or spirulina)

Blend all the ingredients together in a blender.

Vega One Natural and Ginger Recovery Drink

alkaline-forming   antioxidants   calcium   electrolytes   essential fats   iron   phytonutrients

2 large Medjool dates
1 cup water
1 cup coconut water
1 tbsp sprouted buckwheat groats (or substitute cooked)
1 medium banana
1 scoop Vega One Natural
½ tbsp grated fresh ginger

Blend all the ingredients together in a blender.

Pineapple Recovery Drink

alkaline-forming　　calcium　　electrolytes　phytonutrients　　raw

2 large Medjool dates
½ cup chopped fresh pineapple
2 cups water
1 tbsp hemp protein
1 tbsp ground chia
2 tbsp sprouted buckwheat groats (or substitute cooked)
1 tsp ground dulse flakes
1 tsp maca
1 tsp greens powder (chlorella or spirulina)

Blend all the ingredients together in a blender.

Energy Bars

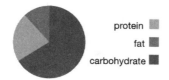

protein
fat
carbohydrate

These bars provide fast and sustained energy, and they are easy and quick to prepare—no cooking required. The only equipment you need is a food processor. In sharp contrast to traditional energy bars, these are true high net-gain food that provides nourishment for sustainable energy. I have made these bars for myself since the mid-1990s. In fact, the recipes that follow are the basis of the Vega Sport Energy Bar that is available in most health food stores and some supermarkets.

The moisture content of berries and dates can vary due to crop conditions, storage methods, and the time elapsed between harvest and final use. If the mixture is too moist to form into a solid bar, add more of the main dry in-gredient. If it is too dry, add more wet ingredients, such as berries, or a small amount of water.

Since I eat a bar or two a day, I make a big batch about once a month. I individually wrap the bars and store them in the freezer. Because these bars stay supple and chewy even when frozen, you can eat them straight out of the freezer. This is a benefit for winter sports also, as many commercial bars freeze solid during skiing or a long winter bike ride. And on a hot day, eating an ice-cold energy bar feels as good as eating ice cream.

You will notice that some of the recipes call for carob powder. It is possible to get raw carob powder, but its flavor is quite weak. So I often use the roasted version. Another alternative is raw chocolate, but it is harder to find and it also contains a bit of caffeine. So, I tend to stick with roasted carob powder for healthy chocolate flavor. Carob is actually a fruit and is therefore quite high in trace minerals.

Energy Bar Procedure Process all ingredients in a food processor until desired texture is reached. If you like a bar with crunch and texture, blend for less time. If you prefer a smooth bar, process longer. If I'm making them specifically for long training rides or for use during physical activity, I blend them smoother, since this helps reduce the amount of energy required for chewing.

Once you've finished processing, remove mixture from processor and put on a clean surface. To shape, flatten mixture with your hands. Cover with cellophane or waxed paper. Roll out with a rolling pin to desired bar thickness. Cut into bars. Or form the mixture into a brick and cut as though you were slicing bread. Let the bars dry for a bit before wrapping and freezing, so they become easier to handle.

Each of these recipes makes approximately 12 bars weighing 50 grams each.

Banana Fig Cinnamon Energy Bar

electrolytes   essential fats   raw

¾ cup soaked dried figs
2 tsp cinnamon
½ tsp nutmeg
1 small banana
½ cup sprouted buckwheat groats (or substitute cooked)
Sea salt to taste
2 tbsp hemp seeds

Process everything except the hemp seeds in a food processor. Once you have cut the bars, sprinkle them with the seeds.

Banana Ginger Energy Bar

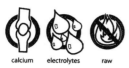

calcium   electrolytes   raw

A refreshingly tasty, crisp bar with lots of nutrients and ginger to help fight inflammation.

¾ cup Medjool dates
2 tbsp grated fresh ginger
1 small banana
½ cup sunflower seeds
¼ cup hemp protein
¾ cup sprouted buckwheat groats (or substitute cooked)
Sea salt to taste
2 tbsp unhulled sesame seeds

Process everything except the sesame seeds in a food processor. Once you have cut the bars, sprinkle them with the seeds.

Carob Strawberry Energy Bar

antioxidants　electrolytes　essential fats　phytonutrients　raw

1 cup Medjool dates (or substitute soaked dried dates)
¼ cup raw carob powder (or substitute roasted carob powder)
¼ cup hemp protein
¼ cup chia
¼ cup strawberries
¼ cup ground flaxseed
¼ cup sunflower seeds
½ tsp lemon zest
1 tsp fresh lemon juice
Sea salt to taste
½ cup sprouted buckwheat groats (or substitute cooked) (optional)
½ cup frozen strawberries

Process everything except the buckwheat groats and frozen strawberries in a food processor. After processing, work in buckwheat groats and frozen strawberries with your hands, then shape and cut as usual.

Spicy Carob Banana Energy Bar

calcium　　electrolytes　　essential fats　　raw

This bar has chocolate flavor with a bit of a bite.

　　¾ cup Medjool dates
　　½ jalapeño pepper
　　1 small banana
　　½ cup sprouted buckwheat groats (or substitute cooked)
　　¼ cup raw carob powder (or substitute raw cacao nibs or
　　　　roasted carob powder)
　　¼ cup chia
　　¼ cup macadamia nuts
　　Sea salt to taste
　　2 tbsp unhulled sesame seeds

Process everything except the sesame seeds in a food processor. Once you have cut the bars, sprinkle them with the seeds.

Green Apple Almond with Greens Energy Bar

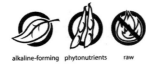

alkaline-forming phytonutrients   raw

This bar has a more traditional flavor but with the health benefits of a nutrient-dense raw bar.

 1 cup Medjool dates
 2 tsp cinnamon
 1 tbsp greens powder (chlorella or spirulina)
 1 small Granny Smith apple, cored
 ½ cup sprouted buckwheat groats (or substitute cooked)
 ¼ cup hemp protein
 ¼ cup soaked raw almonds
 Sea salt to taste

Process everything in a food processor. Cut into bars of desired shape and size.

NON-SPORT-SPECIFIC RECIPES

Apple Cinnamon Chia Granola (Nut-Free)

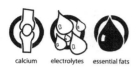

calcium   electrolytes   essential fats

Nutrient-packed and easy to digest, this cereal is a good fuel option a few hours before a workout or soon after to help recovery.

> 1 cup steel-cut oats
> ½ cup hemp protein
> ½ cup ground chia
> 1 cup sunflower seeds
> ½ cup unhulled sesame seeds
> ½ apple, diced
> 1½ tsp cinnamon
> ¼ tsp nutmeg
> ¼ tsp dried and ground stevia leaf
> ¼ tsp sea salt
> ¼ cup Vega Antioxidant EFA Oil Blend (or substitute hemp oil)
> ¼ cup molasses
> 2 tbsp apple juice

Preheat the oven to 250°F. Mix the dry ingredients. Blend the liquid ingredients to a smooth texture, then add the liquid ingredients to the dry. Mix well. Spread on a baking tray lightly coated with oil. Bake for 1 hour. Let cool, then break up into small clusters.

You will notice that I suggest to bake this granola at 250°F instead of the traditional 350°F. This is to prevent the EFAs in the hemp and chia from converting to trans fats.

MAKES ABOUT 4 CUPS OR 5 SERVINGS.

Ginger Pear Chia Granola

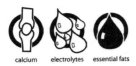

calcium   electrolytes   essential fats

This unique granola has inflammation-reducing properties and a tasty zing of ginger.

    1 cup steel-cut oats
    ½ cup hemp protein
    ½ cup ground chia
    ½ cup unhulled sesame seeds
    1 cup chopped almonds
    ½ pear, diced
    ¼ tsp dried and ground stevia leaf
    ¼ tsp sea salt
    ¼ cup hemp oil
    ¼ cup molasses
    2 tbsp apple juice
    ½ tbsp grated or finely chopped fresh ginger

Preheat the oven to 250°F. Mix the dry ingredients. Blend the liquid ingredients to a smooth texture, then add the liquid ingredients to the dry. Mix well. Spread on a baking tray. Bake for 1 hour. Let cool, then break up into small clusters.

MAKES ABOUT 4 CUPS OR 5 SERVINGS.

Blueberry Pancakes

antioxidants essential fats phytonutrients

These pancakes are an ideal sustainable energy breakfast on the morning of a long bout of exercise such as a bike ride or a hike.

1 cup buckwheat flour
4 scoops Vega Protein & Greens (natural flavor)
2 tsp baking powder
1 tsp cinnamon
½ tsp nutmeg
1 banana
1½ cups water
½–¾ cup blueberries
½ cup buckwheat groats, sprouted or cooked
Coconut oil for frying

In a bowl, mix together buckwheat flour, Vega Protein & Greens, baking powder, cinnamon, and nutmeg.

In a food processor, process banana and water while slowly adding dry ingredients. Process until mixture is smooth. Stir in blueberries and buckwheat groats.

Lightly oil a pan with coconut oil and put on medium heat. Pour in batter to make pancakes and cook for about 5 minutes or until bubbles begin to appear. Flip and cook for another 5 minutes. Since these pancakes contain essential fatty acids that are destroyed at high heat, they are cooked at a lower temperature than traditional pancakes and therefore take a bit longer to cook.

MAKES 2 LARGE SERVINGS.

Collard Greens Buckwheat Wrap

alkaline-forming   antioxidants   calcium   electrolytes   essential fats   iron   phytonutrients   raw

These wraps are packed with nutrition from a variety of sources. Instead of using a typical flour wrap, which would be acid-forming and a low net-gain food, collard greens add a high quality of minerals, are easy to digest, and are packed with blood-building chlorophyll.

1 leaf collard green
1 avocado, diced
2 Roma tomatoes, sliced
1 English cucumber, sliced
1 medium beetroot, grated
2 strips dulse, torn to desired size
1 cup soaked buckwheat groats (or substitute cooked)
2 tbsp Agave Mustard Dressing or Pumpkin Seed Pesto (recipes on page 178)

Place all ingredients except dressing on the leaf of collard, avoiding the edges. Drizzle with dressing and roll up. Cut into desired length. Depending on the size of leaf, this is usually enough for 3 wraps.

Coconut Lime Curry Chickpea Stir-Fry

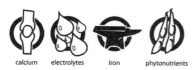

calcium   electrolytes   iron   phytonutrients

Protein-rich and alkalizing, this electrolyte-packed main course is filling yet easily digested. The addition of natural anti-inflammatory ingredients such as turmeric enhances soft tissue repair.

  1 tbsp coconut oil
  1 tbsp grated or finely chopped fresh ginger
  3 cloves garlic, minced
  ½ large red onion, cut lengthwise into thin strips
  1½ cups chopped cauliflower
  1 cup chopped broccoli florets
  1 cup bite-size torn spinach
  ½ tsp curry
  ½ tsp turmeric
  ¼ tsp ground cumin
  ¼ mild chili pepper, finely sliced (or substitute ½ tsp dried chili flakes)
  1 cup cooked chickpeas
  1 cup coconut milk
  1 tbsp fresh lime juice
  ½ cup chopped fresh cilantro

Heat frying pan to medium-high. Add the coconut oil, ginger, and garlic. Lightly stir-fry. Turn heat to medium-low. Add the vegetables, curry, turmeric, cumin, chili pepper, chickpeas, and coconut milk. Cover and cook for 5 minutes. Add the lime juice and cilantro. Serve with sprouted quinoa or buckwheat. Brown rice also works nicely.

MAKES ABOUT 4 SMALL SERVINGS.

Pumpkin Seed Pesto

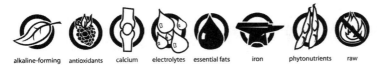

alkaline-forming   antioxidants   calcium   electrolytes   essential fats   iron   phytonutrients   raw

4 cups raw spinach

2 tbsp pumpkin seeds

2 cloves garlic

4 tbsp Vega Antioxidant EFA Oil Blend (or substitute hemp oil or flaxseed oil)

4 tbsp balsamic vinegar

2 tbsp fresh parsley (optional)

Process ingredients in a food processor to desired texture.
Will keep in an open container in the fridge for about 10 days.

Agave Mustard Dressing

antioxidants   essential fats

4 tbsp Vega Antioxidant EFA Oil Blend (or substitute hemp oil)

2 tbsp agave nectar

1 tbsp apple cider vinegar*

1 tbsp Dijon mustard

Sea salt to taste

Combine ingredients in a jar or cup. Stir vigorously to blend.

While vinegar is acidic, it is not actually acid-forming. Upon digestion, it will have an alkaline-forming effect. This is also true of citrus fruit.

Frozen Chocolate Brittle

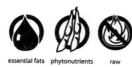

essential fats   phytonutrients   raw

This can serve as a nice frozen snack on a warm day or as pre-workout fuel.

2 tbsp coconut oil
½ scoop Chocolate Vega One
1 tbsp chia (or substitute hemp seeds)
Vega Antioxidant EFA Oil Blend (or substitute hemp oil or flaxseed oil)
    for coating

Heat the coconut oil in a pot on low heat, just until it becomes liquid. Stir in the Vega and chia. Lightly coat the plate with Vega Antioxidant EFA Oil Blend. Pour mixture onto the plate and put in the freezer for about 90 minutes. Remove from the freezer and cut or break into chunks.

For flavor variety, add 1 tsp of lemon, orange, or lime zest and a small amount of sea salt; or a pinch of cayenne; or 1 tbsp agave nectar.

MAKES 1 OR 2 SERVINGS, DEPENDING ON APPETITE.

These smoothies are a few of my favorites and are ideal as a quick, nutrient-dense breakfast or midday snack, or as a drink following a shorter workout such as the 45-minute weight training session. There's even one formulated specially for bedtime.

Chocolate Almond Smoothie

alkaline-forming antioxidants essential fats   iron   phytonutrients

    1 scoop Chocolate Vega One
    2 cups cold water (or 1½ cups water plus 1 cup ice)
    1 banana
    ½ cup blueberries
    ¼ cup soaked raw almonds or almond butter

Blend all the ingredients together in a blender.

MAKES 1 TO 2 SERVINGS, DEPENDING ON APPETITE.

Ginger Pear Smoothie

alkaline-forming antioxidants essential fats   iron   phytonutrients

    1 scoop Vega One Natural
    2 cups cold water (or 1½ cups water plus 1 cup ice)
    1 banana
    ½ pear
    1 tbsp grated fresh ginger

Blend all the ingredients together in a blender.

MAKES 1 TO 2 SERVINGS, DEPENDING ON APPETITE.

Tropical Smoothie

alkaline-forming   antioxidants   essential fats   iron   phytonutrients

1 serving Vega Protein and Greens
2 cups cold water (or 1½ cups water plus 1 cup ice)
1 banana
½ mango (fresh, or 1 cup frozen)
½ cup pineapple

Blend all the ingredients together in a blender.

MAKES 1 TO 2 SERVINGS, DEPENDING ON APPETITE.

Pre-Sleep HGH-Releasing Smoothie

alkaline-forming   electrolytes   essential fats   iron   phytonutrients

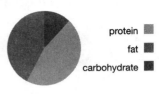

protein
fat
carbohydrate

This smoothie is low in starch and sugar, has plenty of high-quality fat and complete protein, and is rich in L-glutamine (from pea protein), L-arginine, and L-lysine (from walnuts and pine nuts). Because of this, it will enable the body to relax before bed as well as educe the production of HGH, which will speed the recovery process, help build lean muscle, and reduce body fat.

1 handful spinach
¼ cup pine nuts
¼ cup walnuts
1 (2-inch) piece cucumber
1 (2-inch) piece celery
Juice from ½ lemon
½ tsp grated fresh ginger
1 scoop Vega Protein & Greens (natural flavor) (or pea protein)
¾ cup water

Blend all ingredients together in a blender.

MAKES 1 SERVING.

SAMPLE MENU PLAN

The following is an example of how to work the recipes in this book into your daily schedule and around your workout for best results. Serving sizes will vary based on your appetite.

Thrive Fitness sample menu plan and exercise schedule for regular workouts

7:00 A.M. Pre-workout snack: whole food energy bar (recipes start on page 168), or half of Vega One Bar

7:30 A.M. Thrive Fitness workout routine

7:45 A.M. Post-workout snack: whole food smoothie (recipes start on page 180), or Vega One on its own, or 1 scoop blended with fruit

11:00 A.M. Late-morning snack: fruit or the other half of Vega One Bar left over from pre-workout snack

12:30 P.M. Lunch: Collard Greens Buckwheat Wrap (recipe on page 176)

3:30 P.M. Mid-afternoon snack: whole food smoothie (recipes start on page 180), or Vega One on its own, or 1 scoop blended with fruit

7:00 P.M. Dinner: big salad of mixed greens, grated carrots, and dressing of your choice

9:00 P.M. Evening snack: raw pumpkin seeds or raw almonds, or Pre-Sleep HGH-Releasing Smoothie

Thrive Fitness sample menu plan and exercise schedule for longer workouts (such as on the weekend)

8:00 A.M. Breakfast: Apple Cinnamon Chia Granola (recipe on page 173)

10:00 A.M. Pre-workout snack: pre-workout drink (recipes start on page 151)

10:30 A.M. Aerobic exercise

Exercise drink: Start sipping on a sport drink 20 minutes into your workout, then sip every 20 minutes, and more frequently if the temperature and humidity are high.

Exercise snack: If your workout exceeds 90 minutes, have one of the next-generation energy gels at about the 45-minute mark (recipes start on page 153).

Post-exercise drink (within 20 minutes): post-workout recovery drink (recipes start on page 163)

Post-exercise drink (between 45 and 90 minutes after): whole food smoothie (recipes start on page 159) or Vega One on its own, or a half-serving blended with fruit (Vega-specific recipes begin on page 155)

When-you-need-it snack: fruit

6 P.M. Dinner: Coconut Lime Curry Chickpea Stir-Fry (recipe on page 177)

SHOPPING LIST

FRESH FRUIT
apples
bananas
dates
lemons
limes
oranges
papayas
pears
pineapples

VEGETABLES
beets
carrots
cauliflower
celery
collard greens
cucumbers
salad greens, mixed
spinach
tomatoes

FROZEN FRUIT
açaí berries
strawberries
other berries

DRIED NUTS AND SEEDS
almonds (raw)
buckwheat
chia
flaxseed
hemp protein
hemp seed
pumpkin seeds
sesame seeds (unhulled)
sunflower seeds

OTHER
agave nectar
chlorella
dates
coconut oil
coconut water
green tea
maca
molasses
oats
sea vegetables
yerba maté

VEGA ONE
Vega Antioxidant EFA Oil Blend
Vega Protein & Greens (natural flavor)

VEGA PRODUCTS

Vega One

I formulated the original Vega Whole Food Health Optimizer as an evolved replica of the smoothie that I first made for myself at the age of 15. I created it to help speed recovery after exercise—a meal and all my supplements in whole food, liquid form. It supplies complete protein, essential fatty acids, probiotics, fiber, enzymes, antioxidants, chlorella, and maca while promoting a slightly alkaline body pH. This commercial version, renamed Vega One, is a whole food powder that can be mixed with water to supply complete nutrition anytime, anywhere.

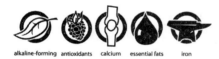
alkaline-forming antioxidants calcium essential fats iron

Vega One Bar

Made from plant-based, whole food, non-GMO ingredients, Vega One Bar is packed with 12 grams protein, 4 grams fiber, and 1 gram omega-3, plus vitamins, minerals, antioxidants, probiotics, and greens.

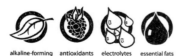
alkaline-forming antioxidants electrolytes essential fats

Vega Protein & Greens

Vega Protein & Greens is a simplified version of Vega One, containing 20 grams complete protein and two servings of greens, for only 110 calories.

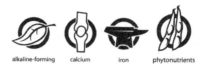
alkaline-forming calcium iron phytonutrients

Vega Antioxidant EFA Oil Blend

This is a synergistic, balanced blend of unrefined, cold-pressed, organic, vegetable oils rich in omega-3 and omega-6 essential fatty acids. A combination of antioxidant-rich superfood oils that include green tea seed, pomegranate seed, and black cumin seed are added to boost nutritional value and antioxidant content. Ideal as a salad dressing base. Numerous recipes for salad dressings can be found in *The Thrive Diet*.

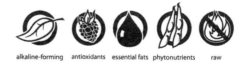
alkaline-forming antioxidants essential fats phytonutrients raw

Vega Snack Bar

These bars are a synergistic combination of non-GMO superfood ingredients, are gluten-free, and contain protein and 1 gram of omega-3.

essential fats phytonutrients

Vega Sport Line

I'd been considering the idea of adding a sport line for several years, and when I began transcribing my sport-specific recipes for this book, I realized it would make sense to offer a convenient, readily available option of each formula. Over the past few years in particular, I've noticed a genuine desire by top professional and recreational athletes alike for a whole food sport nutrition line. The days when athletes accepted low-grade refined products that in no way assist their long-term peak health and performance goals are all but gone.

Vega Sport is a complete, all-natural, plant-based sport performance system specifically developed to help athletes perform at their best. For a holistic ap-proach to sport fueling and recovery, I formulated the Vega Sport performance system in three stages:

- **Prepare** – Fuel with clean, easily digestible energy to burn
- **Sustain** – Clean carbohydrate and electrolytes to enhance performance
- **Recover** – Restock glycogen, reduce inflammation, and speed recovery

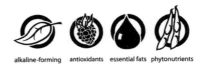

alkaline-forming   antioxidants   essential fats   phytonutrients

For up-to-date Vega news, visit myvega.com.

QUESTIONS AND ANSWERS

8

I don't have much time. Will I be able to incorporate Thrive Fitness into my daily life?

Yes. The foundation of Thrive Fitness can be performed in as little as two and a quarter hours per week. Spending just 45 minutes three times per week will yield impressive results in a matter of weeks. But the best part about the time invested in the program is that you gain it back. Thrive Fitness allows you to build a more capable body that will function more efficiently, thereby reducing the amount of sleep you need and giving you more natural, sustainable energy. On page 47 I explain in detail how Thrive Fitness improves sleep quality so that quantity can be reduced. You will find that once your sleep improves, you will be more alert and more productive.

I don't live near a gym. Can I still take part in Thrive Fitness?

Absolutely. All you need are an inflatable exercise ball, a weighted ball, and push-up stands. You can even do the program without them, but using them will make the exercises more effective.

I've never been able to stick with an exercise program in the past because I have a bad back. Exercise seems to aggravate it. How can I overcome this?

This is a concern for many people. Lower back problems in particular have become ubiquitous in our society for several reasons. For a couple of years, I, too, struggled with a back problem. However, I found that by consistently performing a few simple exercises, I was able to overcome it. I've included a stretching and strengthening program specifically to address lower back concerns. It begins on page 81. I suggest making this part of your daily life if you have had nagging back problems. It will only take about two weeks to notice an improvement. From this point, you can slowly introduce the full Thrive Fitness program.

I enjoy running but seem to get sore shins. Any suggestions?

I know that feeling. About a week after I first began running, I developed shin splints. As I found out, they are among the most common complaints for those new to running. Thankfully, there's a simple way to heal and, better yet, prevent them. Starting on page 84 are exercises specifically designed to strengthen the shin muscles and therefore greatly reduce the risk of developing shin splints. Additionally, I've included a running buildup table on page 85. It uses a systematic approach that incrementally increases mileage no more than 10 percent per week, which will allow your body to adapt to the mileage without overburdening the shins.

How much time will Thrive Fitness take each week?

It can take as little as two hours and 15 minutes per week to do just the basic resistance training program. And up to about six hours if you prefer the comprehensive program that also includes VO_2 max training, repeat-pattern aerobic activity, and continually changing movement activity.

I'm an accomplished athlete. Will Thrive Fitness be able to boost my performance to a new level?

Yes. The program is structured in such a way that it is entirely scalable to your level of fitness. Accomplished strength, power, and endurance athletes can simply boost the intensity and weight during each workout to suit their needs. And since Thrive Fitness is based on the high net-gain principle, all energy exerted, regardless of ability, will yield a high level of return.

I'm a busy executive who would like to boost my energy and reduce the amount of sleep I need in an effort to raise productivity. How can I do this in a natural and sustainable fashion?

Thrive Fitness is geared to boost performance in all facets of life. As fitness levels and therefore muscular efficacy rise, stress and cortisol levels drop. This will enable the body to slip into a deep, efficient form of sleep. People who sleep more efficiently don't need to sleep as long, so they have more time to be productive. Plus they wake up better rested and therefore with more energy, which can of course augment productivity.

I have a family history of Alzheimer's. Is there anything I can do to reduce my risk of getting it?

Yes. Engaging in activities that continually change and therefore require your brain to think about each movement, such as basketball, is said to encourage the construction of neurotransmitters. It is thought that the consistent building of neurotransmitters will reduce the risk of developing neurodegenerative diseases such as Alzheimer's and Parkinson's.

My son has recently been diagnosed with type II diabetes. Will Thrive Fitness help him?

Yes. Regular physical activity and a whole food, nutrient-rich diet such as outlined in this book and *The Thrive Diet* are effective ways to prevent and reverse type II diabetes.

I've always been afraid to begin a weight training program for fear of developing large, bulky muscles. I want toned, lean, functional muscles. Can Thrive Fitness help?

Yes. Thrive Fitness was specifically designed with efficiency for practical purposes. While muscles will grow significantly stronger, they will not become bulky and inhibit functionality.

There are numerous exercise books on the market that promise a drastic visual transformation in a set period of time. Why doesn't Thrive Fitness follow that template?

Thrive Fitness will certainly burn fat and yield impressive visual results. However, these results are simply welcome by-products of the program, not the primary goal. For me, coming from an endurance athlete background, physical activity has always been about efficiency and functionality. As I realized, a strong body that can move with grace and fluidity dramatically improves the overall quality of life. From reduced risk of disease, to increased energy, to improved mental function, Thrive Fitness is about real-world functionality.

Can I work out in the evening instead of the morning?

Yes. Most people find that they prefer to work out in the morning because it helps them start their day feeling good. Also, if you work out first thing, no matter what unfolds throughout the rest of the day, you will have gotten your workout in. However, if your daily schedule lends itself better to an evening workout, that is fine. Whenever you enjoy doing it the most is the best time to do it. Just be mindful of the likelihood that if you go to bed too soon after working out, you may have a more difficult time falling asleep since exercise releases endorphins that help you stay alert.

Can I incorporate only small amounts of the nutrition and Thrive Fitness program and still see results?

Yes. For your nutrition, even one meal or snack a day from the diet can make a noticeable difference over the course of six to eight weeks. Having a fruit smoothie with plant-based protein, essential fatty acids, and fiber for breakfast instead of sugary, starchy cereal is a sensible and easy way to begin.

As for the training program, consistency is one of the most important elements of any physical training program. Because of the physiology of how the body responds to physical exertion and rest, it's important to exercise at least three times a week to experience noticeable results. And, the better your nutrition program, the quicker you will recover from training and therefore the more your body will be able to handle.

I worry that following your dietary advice will cost more money. Will it?

Higher-quality ingredients can cost more than lower-quality ones. I view these food costs as a kind of preventative medicine. The fact that healthy, whole food can prevent sickness from ever occurring is reassuring to me. The good news is that you can cut down on cost if you buy in bulk and/or online.

If the bulk of your diet is healthy, the odds of developing disease later in life are greatly reduced. A major problem now facing senior citizens is the cost of symptom-treating drugs. While in certain areas programs exist to help seniors obtain drugs inexpensively, many simply can't afford them if they are not privy to such assistance. I see it this way: We pay now for higher-quality food or pay later for drugs to treat symptoms caused by poor diet.

Also, people who are healthier don't require as much sleep, have greater energy, better mental clarity, and are physically stronger. This leads to a significant gain in productivity, which saves money too.

For the recipes, are the ingredients hard to find?

I'm pleased to say that an increasing number of major supermarkets now include natural food sections and consequently are an excellent place to find ingredients for the recipes as well as the Top Foods for Peak Performance on page 137. If your local supermarket doesn't carry what you need, you may need to go to a store that specializes in high-quality ingredients, such as a health food store. Many ingredients are also available for purchase in bulk online.

Are the dietary suggestions you give in this book good for children?

Yes. Several organizations devoted to children's health and welfare have reported that there is an undeniable correlation between children's ability to learn and their diet. Processed, sugary foods such as breakfast cereal can cause children to have an energy spike that makes them hyperactive and unable to concentrate. Following a sugar spike, a crash always occurs. During an energy crash, it is incredibly hard for children to focus and retain information presented to them.

I've been told that I have low bone density and may develop osteoporosis. Can Thrive Fitness help?

Yes. Resistance training such as the Thrive Fitness program combined with impact exercise such as walking or run-

ning will help improve bone density by causing ligaments and tendons to pull on the bones, which makes them stronger.

Also, the dietary suggestions in this book and *The Thrive Diet* are alkaline-forming, to prevent bone mass from being broken down in an effort to maintain the blood's neutral acidity level. Refined, processed, denatured foods create an acidic environment within the body. As a survival mechanism, blood draws highly alkaline calcium from the bones to maintain a neutral pH. Over time this leads to weaker bones and possibly to stress fractures in athletes. If not resolved, osteoporosis later in life is likely to transpire.

As a society, we are developing osteoporosis in an earlier stage of life than ever before. This is not due to a lack of dietary calcium as originally thought, but rather to the overconsumption of processed, refined foods that cause calcium to be leached from the bones. *The Thrive Diet* includes a chart showing which foods are acid-forming and which are alkaline-forming.

AFTERWORD

During the late 1800s and early 1900s, newborn elephants were collected, crated, and shipped from their African homeland to the Americas to be trained as circus performers. A young elephant's malleability was coveted most by circus men. Pliability was necessary to "instill" qualities essential to become submissive performers. Upon arrival at their new home under the big top of the circus, the young pachyderms were tethered by a rope around an ankle to a stake in the ground. Day and night for several months, until near exhaustion, the small elephants would struggle to break free, but to no avail. Eventually, the elephants gave up. Their repeated failure instilled in their minds that they were unable to break free. The inability to escape became deeply ingrained. Their will had been broken.

Over the course of a few years, the elephants matured and their mass had grown in excess of five times their arrival weight. As you would expect, along with an increase in size came an increase in strength. Any one of the full-grown elephants could have effortlessly snapped the rope tether. But they didn't. Their previous failed attempts, so deeply rooted, prevented them from even considering escape.

We've all failed at something in the past, and if we haven't, we simply haven't been trying hard enough. But what matters is the present and the future, which we have control over. And by building mental and physical strength, and re-approaching our challenges with justified confidence, success at anything will be easier.

Get stronger. Try again. Thrive.

EXERCISE AND NUTRITION LOGS

Because I've been my own coach since I graduated from high school, I truly learned the value of keeping a detailed training and nutrition log. Every athlete's body responds differently to training. If you include all the pertinent information in a log, over the months, patterns will emerge that magnify even the smallest flaw. With this information, you can make a shift in training focus to fix that flaw.

The log will also allow you to build on successes, since it will reveal exactly what nutrition leads to your best workout performances. From there it's simply a matter of following your log in reverse order and making a note of the workout and nutrition patterns that culminated in your best performance. Conversely, if a performance is subpar, you will have the map that leads to it. But don't feel as though you're a slave to your training log. Record as much or as little information as you feel comfortable with. Filling in at least the basics for each workout and meal will give you a means of tracking your progress. But the more detailed your recording, the greater your ability to use the log as a tool for improvement.

How to Use the Logs

On page 196, you'll find sample and blank training and nutrition log tables. I've also provided a blank log that can be used to record other activities, such as cycling, running, and hiking. As you can see, each table has spaces to record basic information to track progress and, most importantly, reveal patterns.

You may photocopy the template tables to create a logbook. To keep the pages in order, I photocopy several months' worth at a time and have them bound by an office supply store. If you train at a gym, you may want to bring either an individual sheet or your bound logbook with you to record the amount of weight you use for each exercise. Of course, you may prefer to record your training on your smartphone or tablet; for that reason there's a Thrive Fitness app (part of FitPlan) that allows you to track and review your progress. Download information can be found on page 209.

The Week number is pre-printed; it determines the exercises included. Rotation number refers to the number of times you have performed this particular workout as part of the six-week overall training plan. Recording the Day/ Date will help you track progress in a linear fashion.

Time of day started will reveal over time when your body is most likely to perform at its peak. Some people are best suited to morning workouts, while others reach their energy peak later in the day. The Objective of the workout is simply what you have determined the prime focus of your workout to be based on your recorded weakness from the previous training sessions.

Energy level before workout is scored using a five-star scale. If your energy is low, circle one or two stars. If it is excellent, circle five stars. It's normal to have a low-energy day once in a while, but if you find you're consistently circling only just one or two stars, you will need to look at your lifestyle as a whole to determine the cause of your low energy. It is almost always nutrition-related. Following the nutritional guidelines in this book and *The Thrive Diet* will significantly help. Energy level after workout is also based on a five-star system. You will likely find that you regularly circle more stars after your workout than you did before. This is one of the many benefits of exercise; it gives you energy and helps you feel better thanks to endorphin release. Duration of workout is the amount of time it took you to perform your workout.

Weakest link is what you felt held you back from making it a better workout. Did you fade toward the end? Was your breathing choppy? Was your heart rate slow to regulate after the circuit? Were your joints stiff? Did you feel sluggish toward the end of the workout? Once you have determined your weakest link, you can take steps to fix it. A table listing common weak links and how to correct them can be found on pages 206–207.

Strongest element is simply what you felt you excelled at during the workout. Perhaps your strength is a former weak link that you have now overcome.

Under Total Number, Goal is the number of reps recommended and Actual indicates the number you actually performed in that particular workout. This is an important statistic, since it helps you fine-tune the amount of weight ideal for each exercise and indicates whether you fade toward the end of the workout or finish strong. Under Comments, you can record how you felt about the workout and your performance as a whole.

The nutrition section of the log is divided into three main parts. Pre-workout snack is what you eat within an hour of beginning the workout. Post-workout snack is what you eat within an hour of completing the workout. Under Meals/snacks, list any other food you ate that day, and at what time you ate it. The page numbers for the recipes are given in parentheses. Because the quality of each workout is tightly tied to the quality of your nutrition, recording what you ate in detail will shed light on several aspects of workout performance and recovery.

TRAINING AND NUTRITION LOG

Day / Date: _Monday / April 6_

Time of day started: _7:33 A.M._

Objective: _Maintain good form, even toward the end. Focus on breathing._

Energy level before workout: ⟨ * * * * ⟩*

Energy level after workout: ⟨ * * * * ⟩

Duration of workout: _33 min_

Weakest link: _Faltered a bit toward the end._

Strongest element: _Breathing was controlled._

Exercise	Total Number	
	Goal	Actual
Warm up: air squats	30	30
Alternating ball push-up	30	30
Alternating jump ground punch	40	40
Push-ups with leg to opposite knee	40	37
Deep jump squats with elbows thrust up	30	28
Crab craw push-ups	40	40
Skater hops	40	38
V ups with weighted ball	30	30
Surfer spins with full jump	30	28
Chair squat jump	30	27
Mountain climbers	30	30

Comments: _Felt strong at the beginning and throughout most of the workout, but energy dropped off a bit on the last set. Will make sure nutrition is good after workout to ensure high energy for the next one._

Nutrition

Pre-workout snack:　　　Carob Strawberry Energy Bar (recipe on page 170)

Post-workout snack :　　　Chocolate Vega Recovery Drink (recipe on page 164)

Meals / snacks

Time:　　　　　　11:12 a.m.

Description:　　　large pear

Time:　　　　　　12:23 p.m.

Description:　　　Collard Greens Buckwheat Wrap with Pumpkin
　　　　　　　　　Seed Pesto (recipes on pages 176 and 178)

Time:　　　　　　4:22 p.m.

Description:　　　smoothie made with Vega One (recipe suggestions on
　　　　　　　　　pages 180 to 181)

Time:　　　　　　7:10 p.m.

Description:　　　big salad with mixed greens, dulse, sprouts, kale,
　　　　　　　　　with Pumpkin Seed Pesto (recipe on page 178)

Time:　　　　　　9 p.m.

Description:　　　chia with an apple

TRAINING AND NUTRITION LOG

Max Strength / Build / Afterburn

Day / Date: _____

Time of day started: _____

Objective: _____

_____

Energy level before workout: * * * * *

Energy level after workout: * * * * *

Duration of workout: _____

Weakest link: _____

Strongest element: _____

Exercise	Total Number	
	Goal	Actual
Push-ups with stands: favoring one arm at a time	15	
Pistol squats	20	
Lat pull in on ball	15–25	
45 degree angle shoulder press	20	
Bridge to hamstring curl	30	
Triceps press with stands	15	
Step back lunges	20	
Plank leg lift	15	
Superman	20	
Jackknife on ball	30	
Side double crunch	25	

Comments: _____
_____
_____

Nutrition
Pre-workout snack: _____

Post-workout snack: _____

Meals / snacks
Time: _____
Description: _____
_____

Time: _____
Description: _____
_____

Time: _____
Description: _____
_____

Time: _____
Description: _____
_____

Time: _____
Description: _____
_____

TRAINING AND NUTRITION LOG

Strength Conversion / Power / Efficiency

Day / Date: _____

Time of day started: _____

Objective: _____
_____

Energy level before workout: * * * * *

Energy level after workout: * * * * *

Duration of workout: _____

Weakest link: _____

Strongest element: _____

Exercise	Total Number	
	Goal	Actual
Warm up: 30 air squats	30	
Alternating ball push-up	30	
Alternating jump ground punch	40	
Push-ups with leg to opposite knee	40	
Deep jump squats with elbows thrust up	30	
Crab craw push-ups	40	
Skater hops	40	
V ups with weighted ball	30	
Surfer spins with full jump	30	
Chair squat jump	30	
Mountain climbers	30	

Comments: _____
_____
_____

Nutrition

Pre-workout snack: _____

Post-workout snack: _____

Meals / snacks

Time: _____
Description: _____
_____

Time: _____
Description: _____
_____

Time: _____
Description: _____
_____

Time: _____
Description: _____
_____

Time: _____
Description: _____
_____

TRAINING AND NUTRITION LOG

VO$_2$ / Lung Power / Functional Strength

Day / Date: _____

Time of day started: _____

Objective: _____

_____

Energy level before workout: * * * * *

Energy level after workout: * * * * *

Duration of workout: _____

Weakest link: _____

Strongest element: _____

Exercise	Total Number	
5 min warm-up (jogging, walking stairs, jumping jacks, etc.)		
Rotate through circuit 2 times. About 30 minutes, maximum 30 seconds rest between each exercise.		
	Goal	**Actual**
Fast pushup knee to elbow	30	
Bicycling with ball	60	
Alternating plyometric lunge	40	
Roll to cross with arms out	40	
Deep squat with weighted ball throw	25	
In and out with arms parallel on the ball	20	
Jump squat while lifting weighted ball straight out and up	20	
Double crunch	30	
Squat sidekicks	40	
Swooping cobra push-ups	20	
Plank	90 seconds	

Comments: _____
_____
_____

Nutrition

Pre-workout snack: _____

Post-workout snack: _____

Meals / snacks

Time: _____
Description: _____
_____

Time: _____
Description: _____
_____

Time: _____
Description: _____
_____

Time: _____
Description: _____
_____

Time: _____
Description: _____
_____

TRAINING AND NUTRITION LOG

Activity: _____

Day / Date: _____

Time started: _____

Duration: _____

Description: _____
_____
_____
_____
_____
_____
_____
_____

Comments: _____
_____
_____
_____
_____
_____
_____
_____
_____
_____
_____
_____
_____
_____

Nutrition

Pre-activity snack: _____

During activity snack: _____

Post-activity snack: _____

Meals / snacks

Time: _____
Description: _____
_____

Time: _____
Description: _____
_____

Time: _____
Description: _____
_____

Time: _____
Description: _____
_____

Time: _____
Description: _____
_____

Fixing Weak Links

Following is a list of common weak links and their solutions.

Weak link	Solution
Felt sluggish at the beginning.	Do a longer warm-up to get blood flowing better. Until the body gets used to a short warm-up, you may need 10 minutes. Each week, reduce the warm-up by one minute, leveling off at five minutes. Low blood sugar may also be a factor. Make sure to eat a pre-workout snack before each session. Recipes start on page 168.
Faded toward the end of the workout.	This could simply be a matter of the body adapting to the new workload. Once fitness improves over the course of about two weeks, fading toward the end should no longer occur. It could also be nutrition-related. Ensure your nutrition the day prior to your workout is sound.
Stiff and inflamed muscles and joints, inhibited range of motion.	This is likely an indication that your previous workout was more taxing than your body is ready to handle and adapt to at this point. Light stretching can be helpful. Follow the program starting on page 80. A diet rich in alkaline-forming foods such as those outlined in this book and *The Thrive Diet* can play a significant role in the reduction of inflammation and therefore improve range of motion.
Heart rate does not drop or regulate before starting next set.	It is likely that you are still developing fitness. If you continue with the program, within a couple of weeks you will notice your heartbeat regulating quicker. However, if your heart rate regulated quickly for the past two weeks and now it doesn't, it is likely that you are simply tired; your muscles are inefficient due to fatigue. Take a rest for a couple of days and then reintroduce activity.

Weak link	Solution
Poor concentration.	This is likely caused by low blood sugar. Make sure your pre-workout snack is well balanced.
Muscles shake toward the end.	This could simply mean you have worked hard earlier in the workout and your muscles are getting tired. This is not something to worry about.
Muscles twitch or cramp toward the end.	This could be because you are still building fitness. If this is the case, the problem will clear up within two weeks of consistent training. Or it may indicate dehydration, in which case you will need to consume a sport drink that contains electrolytes. Recipes for sport drinks start on page 151. In warmer climates, be sure to sip an electrolyte drink throughout the day to prevent dehydration.
Feel hungry before workout is complete.	If you had your pre-workout snack yet you find that you still get hungry before the workout is complete, you may want to carry an energy gel with you while working out. Recipes start on page 153. You will find that as you get fitter, your body's efficiency will improve and therefore you will not burn fuel as quickly—and thus won't need to refuel as often.

MOBILE APP

To complement the Thrive Fitness program, you may download the mobile app that will allow you to follow my exact training methods while on the go, see each exercise in this book demonstrated, as well as get plant-based performance nutrition tips and detailed meal plans that will help you get the most out of the Thrive Fitness program.

Through Thrive Fitness on Fitplan, you'll also be able to track each of your workouts on the mobile log, and be part of a supportive social community dedicated to your success.

Download the Thrive Fitness Fitplan app at www.fitplan.io.

GLOSSARY

Active meditation Performing repeat-pattern aerobic activity while allowing the mind to wander in a meditative state that is conscious but not focused is referred to as active meditation. It is particularly beneficial for stimulating the right brain and thereby creativity.

Aerobic exercise Aerobic means with oxygen. Any exercise that requires the constant breathing of oxygen to maintain pace is considered aerobic. Running at a moderate pace is an aerobic form of exercise, while sprinting full-out is not. Sprinting is classified as anaerobic, that is, without oxygen.

Anaerobic threshold Sometimes referred to as lactate threshold, anaerobic threshold is the point during intense exercise that lactate starts to accumulate in the bloodstream faster than it can be metabolized. Once this point is reached, intensity must be reduced or endurance will sharply decline.

Antioxidants Antioxidants are the name given to several naturally occurring compounds—vitamin C, vitamin E, selenium, and carotenoids—prized for their cell-protection and cell-regeneration attributes. They help remove body-aging and cancer-causing free radicals from the body.

Biological age fix Biological age fix refers to the time that has passed since the most recent round of cellular regeneration has taken place. It can be reduced by speeding the regeneration process of the body. Complementary stress such as exercise and high-quality food reduce biological age, while uncomplementary stress and refined foods increase it.

Biological debt Biological debt refers to a state the body goes into after energy from stimulation has dissipated. Often brought about by eating refined sugar or drinking coffee to gain short-term energy, biological debt is a state of fatigue.

Catabolic A metabolic state in which a "breaking down" rather than a "building up" occurs in body tissues is referred to as catabolic. This state is most commonly precipitated by stress, and therefore the release of cortisol.

Electrolyte Electrolytes are electricity-conducting salts. Electrolytes in body tissue and blood conduct charges that are essential for muscle contractions, heartbeats, and fluid regulation. Chloride, calcium, magnesium, sodium, and potassium are the chief electrolyte minerals. When too few of these minerals are ingested in food or fluid, muscle cramps and heart palpitations can result. In addition, when too much fluid that does not contain electrolytes is consumed, it can flush out the remaining electrolytes.

Empty foods Also referred to as empty calories, empty foods are heavily processed or refined. With little if any nutritional value, empty foods (often full of starch and sugar) retain their calories, which can lead to quick weight gain and a feeling of never being satisfied.

Fitness capital Once you are fit, you are said to have fitness capital: an abundance of energy, mental clarity, and drive that will raise the odds of success in any chosen pursuit. As with other forms of capital, such as financial or political, fitness capital needs to be spent to be of practical value.

Free radicals These damaging compounds that alter cell membranes and can adversely affect our DNA occur naturally in the body, where they are produced on a daily basis in small amounts. However, as stress increases, so, too, does the production of free radicals. If stress is allowed to persist for an extended period of time, damage done by free radicals leads to cancer and other serious diseases. Free radicals also cause premature signs of aging, including in the skin, when allowed to remain in the system. A reduction of stress through better nutrition combats free radical production. Antioxidants in foods help to rid the body of free radicals by escorting them out of the body.

High net-gain nutrition *Net gain* is the term I use to refer to the usable nutrition the body is left with once food is digested and assimilated. Food that is rich in nutritional components but requires little energy to digest and assimilate can be referred to as high net-gain food. The higher the net-gain of food, the more energy that can be garnered from it.

High-return exercise Exercise that yields a benefit in several forms that is of greater value than the energy put forth can be referred to as high-return exercise. High-return exercise is not just about getting fit and strong, it is also about the mental benefits, namely a boost in creativity and building of neurotransmitters.

Human growth hormone Human growth hormone, often simply referred to as HGH, is what stimulates muscular growth and cell reproduction. It is released during intense exercise and sleep.

Justified confidence Justified confidence is built by addressing a problem that formerly inhibited success. It differs from regular confidence in that to create it, steps have been intentionally taken to address a weak point.

Left brain The hemisphere of the brain that is responsible for systematic, analytical, linear thought.

Mental outsourcing I refer to delegating left-brain jobs that were formerly the responsibility of the brain as mental outsourcing. For example, writing down a to-do list instead of using brain power to try to remember what needs to be done or using a GPS device while driving to find an address instead of trying to remember directions and having to focus on what exit to take. It results in greater mental clarity, from which creativity can take root.

Muscular functionality Muscles that are fit and move with ease while putting minimal strain on the cardiovascular system due to their superior efficiency can be said to have become functional. Strength equals efficiency, which culminates in muscular functionality.

Nutrient-dense Sometimes also referred to as nutrient-rich, these are foods that are unrefined and therefore packed with nutrition. Some foods are inherently more nutrient-dense than others; ones with high levels of antioxidants and an abundance of vitamins and minerals are said to be nutrient-dense.

Phytonutrient A phytonutrient is a plant compound that can offer health benefits independent of its nutritional value. Phytonutrients are not essential for life, but they improve vitality.

Repeat-pattern aerobic activity This type of activity is composed of a pattern of repetitive motion that requires oxygen. For example, running, cycling, and swimming.

Right brain The hemisphere of the brain that is responsible for creative, abstract thought. It can be stimulated with repeat-pattern aerobic activity.

Select information diet You are said to be on a select information diet when you purposefully limit your intake of non-important information with the intent of processing existing information more efficiently. It is particularly useful when trying to maximize the ability of the subconscious to problem solve.

Simple carbohydrate Sometimes referred to as simple sugar, simple carbohydrate is prevalent in most fruits. The body's most usable, and therefore first, choice for fuel, simple carbohydrate is necessary for both mental and physical activity. If the body is not fed foods that contain simple carbohydrates, it will have to convert complex carbohydrates, but that takes extra work and therefore is not a good use of energy. Glucose and fructose, being the primary simple carbohydrates, are the ideal fuel in that they are already in a form that the body can utilize. Plus, digestive enzymes are able to break them down more efficiently than their complex carbohydrate counterparts.

Strength-to-weight ratio The amount of weight able to be lifted in comparison to body weight is known as the strength-to-weight ratio. It is particularly advantageous for endurance athletes to increase this ratio, because becoming stronger will garner no performance improvement if body weight also rises. This is because the extra weight of the muscle will offset the strength gains. Strength-to-weight ratio can be increased by building muscular strength (and therefore efficiency and practical function) while not increasing the size or weight of the muscle.

VO_2 max This is also referred to as maximal oxygen consumption, maximal oxygen uptake, or aerobic capacity. It is the maximum capacity of an individual to transport and utilize oxygen during incremental exercise. Usually performed on a treadmill, a VO_2 max test is considered to be one of the most reliable ways of assessing an individual's fitness level.

Whole food Foods that have had no part removed during processing are known as whole foods. The term is also used to refer to foods that are simply in their natural state, such as fresh, raw fruit and vegetables.

RESOURCES

Beast Burger by Beyond Meat

This truly unique plant-based burger is ideal for athletes. Not only does it have 23 grams of protein per serving, with antioxidants, iron, calcium, vitamins B6, B12, and D, potassium, DHA and ALA omega-3s, it also features the Beyond Nutrient Pack, which aids in muscle recovery. It is gluten-free, soy-free, cholesterol-free, and non-GMO.

    beyondmeat.com

ReFuel

My friend and I created this free app. Simply put: it will advise you when and what to eat and drink to maximize performance. ReFuel syncs with activity trackers to determine your hydration and fuel requirements, based on output, and makes recommendations for you in accordance with my plant-based performance nutrition guidelines. To maximize individual performance, it will advise you what to eat and drink leading up to a workout to ideally fuel; during a workout to ensure maximum sustainability; and immediately following a workout to optimize performance and reduce inflammation and recovery time.

    refuelapps.com

**Sports Nutrition and Elite Sports Nutrition online courses
with Matthew Kenney and Brendan Brazier**

Based on my book *The Thrive Diet*, with the help of a live instructor, I'll guide you through tailored plant-based meal plans related to specific athletic goals of strength training, endurance training, or optimal weight management. I'll also take you through customized, elite athletic training plans, complemented with nutrient-dense, whole food recipes.

    matthewkenneycuisine.com/education

The People's Movement

The People's Movement creates eco-hip footwear and accessories that stand for reduction of single-use plastic. I've partnered with MOVMT to create an affordable high-performance training shoe, made from hemp and up-cycled plastic.

thepeoplesmovement.com/brazier

Thrive Foods Direct

Based on recipes from my book *The Thrive Diet*, you may now have organic, plant-based, gluten-free, whole food meals delivered to your door, anywhere in the United States.

thrivefoodsdirect.com

Thrive Forward Web Series

I developed this in-depth free web series to help people assess their specific needs and customize a program to help them live to their full potential. Includes over 40 videos, meal plans, recipes, and downloadable material.

thriveforward.com

Thrive Market

Thrive Market is an online membership community that allows you to get premium natural and organic food at wholesale prices, anywhere in the United States. And for every membership sold, one is given to an American family in need, to ensure that high-quality food isn't only for the wealthy.

Thrivemarket.com

THRIVE on VyRT

I've teamed up with VyRT, the commercial-free live video-streaming service created by Oscar winner and 30 Seconds to Mars frontman, Jared Leto.

Thrive is a plant-based performance nutrition show where you'll get up close and personal with today's top performers and gain an inside look at how elite bodies and minds are fueled, plus learn the mental and physical techniques they've used to get on top, and stay there. My guests include professional athletes, Olympic champions, elite fitness trainers, world-renowned musicians, top tech entrepreneurs, and more.

vyrt.com/live/thrive

Vega

In 2004, we launched a commercial version of the blender drink that I had made for myself the previous few years while racing Ironman triathlons professionally. It was packed with multi-source plant-based protein, omega-3s, maca, chlorella, enzymes, probiotics, vitamins, and minerals. We called it Vega Complete Whole Food Health Optimizer. Since then, we renamed it Vega One. Following Vega One, we've brought out several other products, including a variety of bars and an entire Sport line. For complete info, recipes, and meal plans, visit:

myvega.com

ZoN Fitness

Check out ZoN Fitness for quality home fitness equipment. I've partnered with them to create plant-based recipes, meal plans, and other downloadable material.

zonfitness.com

Social media handles:

T: @brendan_brazier
I: @brendanbrazier
F: facebook.com/brendanbrazier

REFERENCES

Adlercreutz, H. "Western Diet and Western Diseases: Some Hormonal and Biochemical Mechanisms and Associations," supplement *Scandinavian Journal of Clinical and Laboratory Investigation* 201(1990): 3–23.

Burke, E. R. *Optimal Muscle Recovery*. New York: Avery, 1999.

Cao, G., et al. "Antioxidant Capacity of Tea and Common Vegetables." *Journal of Agricultural and Food Chemistry* 4, no. 34: (1996): 26–31.

———. "Increases in Human Plasma Antioxidant Capacity after Consumption of Controlled Diets High in Fruit and Vegetables." *American Journal of Clinical Nutrition* 68 (1998): 1081–1087.

Centers for Disease Control and Prevention. "Risk Factor for Meeting Recommended Guidelines for Moderate Physical Activity." Behavioral Risk Factor Surveillance System, 2003. Available at http://apps.nccd.cdc.gov/brfss/list.asp?cat=PA&yr=2003&qkey=4418&state=All.

———. "Obesity trends among U.S. adults. Behavioral Risk Factor Surveillance System." (1985–2003). Available at www.cdc.gov/nccdphp/dnpa/obesity/trend/maps.

Colgan, M. *Optimum Sports Nutrition: Your Competitive Edge*. New York: Advanced Research Press, 1993.

———. *Hormonal Health*: *Nutritional and Hormonal Strategies for Emotional Well-Being and Longevity*. Vancouver: Apple, 1995.

Conrad, C. *Hemp for Health: The Medicinal and Nutritional Uses of Cannabis Sativa*. Rochester, VT: Inner Traditions, 1997.

Consumers Union Education Services. *Captive Kids: A Report on Commercial Pressures on Kids at School*. Yonkers, NY: Consumers Union, 1998.

Cordain, L. *The Paleo Diet: Lose Weight and Get Healthy by Eating the Food You Were Designed to Eat*. New York: Wiley, 2001.

Coulstron, A. M. "The Role of Dietary Fats in Plant-Based Diets," supplement, *American Journal of Clinical Nutrition* 70 (1999): 512S–515S.

De Kloet, E. R. "Corticosteroids, Stress, and Aging." *Annals of New York Academy of Sciences* 663 (1992): 358.

Ferrandiz, M. L., et al. "Anti-Inflammatory Activity and Inhibition of Arachidonic Acid Metabolism by Flavonoids." *Agents and Actions* 32 (1991): 283–288.

Hart, A. *Adrenaline and Stress: The Exciting New Breakthrough That Helps You Overcome Stress Damage.* Rev. ed. Dallas: Word Publishing, 1995.

Hayflick, L. *How and Why We Age.* New York: Ballantine, 1994.

Health Canada. *Canadian Guidelines for Body Weight Classification in Adults.* Catalogue H49–179. Ottawa: Health Canada, 2003.

Howard Hughes Medical Institute. "Controlling Brain Wiring with the Flick of a Chemical Switch." April 7, 2005. Available at www.hhmi.org/news/ginty2.html.

Kikuzaki, H., Y. Kawasaki, and N. Nakatani. "Structure of Antioxidative Compounds in Ginger." *American Chemistry Society Symposium Series* 574 (1994): 237–243.

Kraemer, W. J., et al. "Effects of Heavy-Resistance Training on Hormonal Response Patterns in Younger and Older Men." *Journal of Applied Physiology* 87, no. 3 (1999): 982–992.

Krebs-Smith, S. M., et al. "The Effects of Variety in Food Choices on Dietary Quality." *Journal of the American Dietetic Association* 87, no. 7 (1987): 896–903.

Kusnecov, A. and B. S. Rabin. "Stressor-Induced Alterations of Immune Function: Mechanisms and Issues." *International Archives of Allergy and Immunology* 105, no. 2 (1994): 107–121.

Lardinois, C. K. "The Role of Omega-3 Fatty Acids on Insulin Secretion and Insulin Sensitivity." *Medical Hypotheses* 24, no. 3 (1997): 243–248.

Leibowitz, S., et al. "Insulin Plays Role in Controlling Fat Craving." *Newswire.* News from the Rockefeller University, New York, July 27, 1995.

Levenstein, Harvey. *Paradox of Plenty: A Social History of Eating in Modern America.* New York: Oxford University Press, 1993.

Ley, B. M. *Maca: Adaptogen and Hormonal Regulator.* Detroit Lakes: BL Publications, 2003.

———. *Chlorella: The Ultimate Green Food.* Detroit Lakes: BL Publications, 2003.

Moon, Karen. "Healthy Employees Can Result in a Healthy Bottom Line." *The Journal Record* (Oklahoma City). October 4, 2008.

National Center for Health Statistics. "Prevalence of overweight and obesity among adults: United States, 1999–2002." National Health and Nutrition Examination Survey. Available at www.cdc.gov/nchs/data/hestat/obese/obese99.htm.

News-Medical.Net. "Exercise Can Help Brain Healing Process." Medical Research News. June 2, 2004. Available at www.news-medical.net/?id=2144.

———. "Exercise Protects Brain Cells Affected by Parkinson's." Medical Research News. October 24, 2004. Available at www.news-medical.net/?id=5782.

Nick, G. L. "Detoxification Properties of Low-Dose Phytochemical Complexes Found within Select Vegetables." *Journal of American Nutraceutical Association* 5, no. 4 (2002): 34–44.

Oster, G., D. Thompson, J. Edelsberg, A. P. Bird, and G. A. Colditz. "Lifetime Health and Economic Benefits of Weight Loss among Obese Persons." *American Journal of Public Health* 89 (1999): 1536–1542.

Pert, C. *Molecules of Emotions: Why You Feel the Way You Feel.* New York: Touchstone, 1999, 22–23.

Pratt, M. L., C. A. Macera, and G. Wang. "Higher Direct Medical Costs Associated with Physical Inactivity." *The Physician and Sportsmedicine* 28, no. 10 (2000): 63–70.

Richardson, J. H., T. Palmenton, and H. Chenan. "The Effect of Calcium on Muscle Fatigue." *Journal of Sports Medicine and Physical Fitness* 20 (1980): 149–151.

Roux, L., and C. Donaldson. "Economics and Obesity: Costing the Problem or Evaluating Solutions?" *Obesity Research* 12, no. 2 (2004): 173–179.

Russo-Neustadt, A. A., R. C. Beard, Y. M. Huang, and C. W. Cotman. "Physical Activity and Antidepressant Treatment Potentiate the Expression of Specific Brain-Derived Neurotrophic Factor Transcripts in the Rat Hippocampus." *Neuroscience* 101 (2000): 305–312.

Simopoulos, A. P. "Essential Fatty Acids in Health and Chronic Disease" supplement, *American Journal of Clinical Nutrition* 70 (1990): 560S–569S.

Somer, E. *Food and Mood: The Complete Guide to Eating Well and Feeling Your Best.* New York: Holt, 1999.

Stoll, A. L. *The Omega-3 Connection.* New York: Simon & Schuster, 2001.

Teitelbaum, J. E., W. A. Walker. "Nutritional Impact of Pre- and Probiotics as Protective Gastrointestinal Organisms." *Annual Review of Nutrition* 22 (2002): 107–138.

Van Cauter, E., and G. Copinschi. "Interrelationships Between Growth Hormone and Sleep" supplement B, *Growth Hormone and IGH Research* (April 2000): S57–62.

Viru, A. *Hormones in Muscular Activity.* Boca Raton, FL: CRC Press, 1985.

Wang, G., Z. J. Zheng, G. Heath, C. Macera, M. Pratt, and D. Buchner. "Economic Burden of Cardiovascular Disease Associated with Excess Body Weight in U.S. Adults." *American Journal of Preventative Medicine* 23, no. 1 (2002): 1–6.

Wilson, J. L. *Adrenal Fatigue: The 21st-Century Stress Syndrome.* Petaluma, CA: Smart Publications, 2002.

Wood, R. *The New Whole Foods Encyclopedia: A Comprehensive Resource for Healthy Eating.* New York: Penguin, 1999.

Wurtman, J. J., and S. Suffers. *The Serotonin Solution.* New York: Ballantine, 1997.

Youdim, K. A., A. Martin, and J. A. Joseph. "Essential Fatty Acids and the Brain: Possible Health Implications." *International Journal of Developmental Neuroscience* 18 (2000): 383–399.

Young, V. R., and P. L. Pellett. "Plant Proteins In Relation to Human Protein and Amino Acid Nutrition." *American Journal of Clinical Nutrition* 59, no. 5 (1994): 1203S–1212S.

INDEX

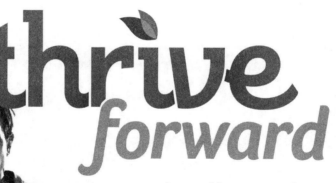

thrive forward

Developed by Brendan Brazier, Thrive Forward is a **FREE**, personalized online guide to help transform your health and performance through plant-based nutrition.

THRIVE FORWARD CONTENT INCLUDES:

 Videos

 Tips & tricks

 eBooks

Reference Lists

 Recipes

 Articles

Thrive Forward has all the tools you need to make small, easy changes to transform your life.

SIGN UP FOR FREE AT
thriveforward.com

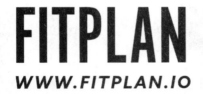
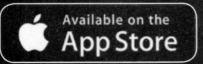
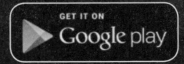

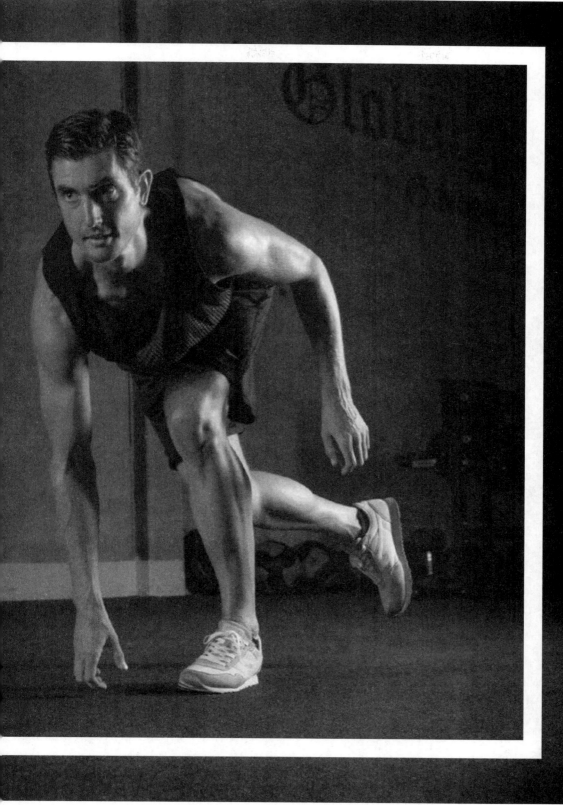